MW00714694

Study Guide

Michele T. Martin
Wesleyan College

Patricia J. Conrod
University of British Columbia

Abnormal Psychology

Canadian Edition

Thomas F. Oltmanns

Robert E. Emery

Steven Taylor

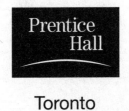

Prentice Hall

Toronto

ISBN 0-13-042509-5

Acquisitions Editor: Jessica Mosher
Developmental Editor: Lise Dupont
Production Editor: Avivah Wargon
Production Coordinator: Wendy Moran

1 2 3 4 5   06 05 04 03 02

Printed and bound in Canada.

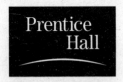

Prentice
Hall

TABLE OF CONTENTS

PREFACE

Your instructor has selected an excellent textbook on abnormal psychology. The material presented in your text emphasises both the latest information on clinical disorders and the description of major research paradigms used in this area of study. We hope that you will enjoy learning about this fascinating area of psychology.

As you read through your textbook, note that all of the chapters are organised similarly. Every chapter begins with an overview of the types of disorders that will be introduced in that chapter. A description of the typical symptoms and associated features of the disorders is then presented, followed by a review of major classification issues, including current diagnostic criteria for each disorder. A discussion of epidemiological aspects of the disorders follows, focusing on incidence, prevalence, and gender and cross-cultural differences. Etiological factors that contribute to the development and manifestation of these disorders are then presented. Finally, treatment approaches to the disorders are discussed. Each chapter concludes with a chapter summary. Being aware of this broad organisational outline will help you organise and study the chapter material more efficiently.

Throughout the chapters, you will notice key terms that are italicised. The definitions of these terms are important for you to know. At the end of each chapter of your textbook, you will find a chapter summary. This summary is a detailed abstract of your chapter, and it will be helpful if you review each summary before working on the questions included in this study guide.

This study guide is organised to maximise your efficient review and comprehension of the material presented in your textbook. Each chapter begins with a **Chapter Outline** that parallels the outline featured in your textbook. Studying this outline will help you organise your review of the material presented in your text. The **Learning Objectives** highlight specific ideas, concepts, and issues that you should understand. The **Key Terms — Matching** tests whether you can match the italicised items included in your textbook with their definitions. The **Names You Should Know — Matching** tests whether you can match the names of people with the important contributions they have made in that area of study. The **Review of Concepts — Fill in the Blank and True/False** and the **Multiple Choice Questions** will help you determine how well you have mastered the oncepts and information presented in your text. In certain chapters, the **Understanding Research — Fill in the Blank** will help you to review the research studies and issues described in detail in the text. Finally, answering the **Brief Essay** questions will help you integrate information that has been presented throughout the chapter. In addition to answering these essay questions, it is important to review the critical thinking questions at the end of each chapter in your text.

We hope that you will find this study guide to be a valuable resource for your work this semester. Reviewing all of the sections and completing all of the exercises for each chapter should be very helpful as you prepare for exams. Good luck and enjoy your course!

CHAPTER 1
EXAMPLES AND DEFINITIONS OF ABNORMAL BEHAVIOUR

Chapter Outline

I. Abnormal Psychology: An Overview
    A. Clinical Science
    B. The Uses and Limitations of Case Studies

II. What is Abnormal Behaviour?
    A. Recognizing Symptoms of Disorder
    B. Defining Abnormal Behaviour
        1. Harmful Dysfunction
        2. DSM-IV Definition
        3. Cultural Considerations

III. Boundaries of Abnormal Behaviour
    A. Dimensions Versus Categories
    B. Frequency in Community Populations
    C. Cross-Cultural Comparisons
    D. Research Close-Up: Cross-Cultural Study of Abnormal Behaviour

IV. Causes and Treatment of Abnormal Behaviour
    A. Nature and Nurture
    B. Systems of Influence
    C. Treatment Methods
    D. The Mental Health Professions

V. Psychopathology in Historical Context
    A. The Greek Tradition in Medicine
    B. The Creation of the Asylum
    C. Lessons from the History of Psychopathology
    D. Canadian Focus: Dr. Ewen Cameron and the Allan Memorial Institute
    E. Research Methods: The Null Hypothesis and the Burden of Proof

VI. Goals of This Book

Learning Objectives

After reviewing the material presented in this chapter, you should be able to:

1. Know a basic definition of abnormal psychology.

2. Understand the scientist-practitioner model.

3. Consider the three primary criteria of abnormality (subjective distress, statistical infrequency, and maladaptiveness) in terms of their strengths and weaknesses.

4. Distinguish the dimensional approach to abnormality from the categorical approach.

5. Know the terms epidemiology, incidence, and prevalence.

6. Describe the nature-nurture controversy in abnormal psychology and explain why it should not be a controversy since nature and nurture interact.

7. Compare the individual, social, and biological systems of influence.

8. Define and understand the advantages and disadvantages of biological reductionism.

9. Understand that changes due to a certain form of treatment do not prove causality.

10. Recognize the differences between a demonological and a natural scientific approach to psychopathology.

11. Know the historical development within institutional treatment of mental disorders.

12. Understand the importance of recognizing cultural issues and using scientific research to establish the validity of approaches to psychopathology.

13. Appreciate the "conservative" approach in research, leading to a reluctance to reject the null hypothesis until evidence establishes the validity of a new theory.

Key Terms — Matching #1

The following terms related to abnormal psychology are important to know. To test your knowledge, match the following terms with their definitions. Answers are listed at the end of the chapter.

a. Psychology
b. Abnormal psychology
c. Scientist-practitioner model
d. Case study
e. Comorbidity
f. Psychopathology
g. Psychosis
h. Delusion
i. Disorganized speech
j. Bulimia nervosa

k. Categorical approach
l. Dimensional approach
m. Threshold model
n. Dichotomous decision
o. Epidemiology
p. Incidence
q Prevalence
r. Lifetime prevalence
s. Etiology

1. ____ the presence of more than one condition within the same period of time
2. ____ the scientific study of behaviour, cognition, and emotion
3. ____ the scientific study of the frequency and distribution of disorders within a population
4. ____ an idiosyncratic belief, not shared by other members of the society, that is rigidly held despite its preposterous nature
5. ____ a symptom often found in schizophrenia of speech that is odd and difficult to comprehend; a problem with the form of speech rather than content
6. ____ a view of classification based on the assumption that behaviour is distributed on a continuum from normal to abnormal, and that differences between forms of mental disorder are quantitative rather than qualitative
7. ____ the total number of active cases of a disorder present in a population during a specific period of time
8. ____ the total proportion of people in a population who have been affected by the disorder at some point in their lives
9. ____ a descriptive presentation of the psychological problems of one particular person
10. ____ emphasizes the integration of science and clinical practice
11. ____ a state of being profoundly out of touch with reality
12. ____ the causes of a disorder
13. ____ required in making a diagnosis; determining whether a particular person fits a diagnostic category rather than the degree to which they possess a characteristic
14. ____ a form of eating disorder characterized by bingeing and purging
15. ____ the manifestations of, and study of the causes of, mental disorders
16. ____ a view of classification based on the assumption that there are qualitative differences between normal and abnormal behaviour and between different types of abnormal behaviour

17. ____ the application of psychological science to the study of mental disorders
18. ____ a combination of dimensional and categorical approaches to classification stating that people can exhibit characteristics of a disorder without any harm to their adjustment until they pass a critical threshold, where there is a dramatic increase in the number of problems they encounter
19. ____ the number of new cases of a disorder that appear in a population during a specific time

Key Terms — Matching #2

The following terms related to abnormal psychology are important to know. To test your knowledge, match the following terms with their definitions. Answers are listed at the end of the chapter.

1. Formal thought disorder
2. Insanity
3. Not guilty by reason of insanity
4. Nervous breakdown
5. Descriptive psychopathology
6. Syndrome
7. Schizophrenia
8. Provincial boards of examiners
9. Harmful dysfunction
10. Diagnostic and Statistical Manual of Mental Disorders (DSM)
11. Nature-nurture controversy
12. Biopsychosocial model
13. Psychopharmacology
14. Psychotherapy
15. Culture
16. Moral treatment movement
17. Psychiatry
18. Experimental hypothesis
19. Null hypothesis
20. Clinical psychology
21. Social work
22. Professional Counselors
23. Marriage and Family Therapy (MFT) counselors
24. Psychiatric Nursing
25. Psychosocial Rehabilitation

a. ____ a mental disorder characterized by psychotic symptoms, disorganized speech, and emotional flatness and withdrawal
b. ____ any new prediction made by a researcher
c. ____ a group of symptoms that appear together and are assumed to represent a specific type of disorder
d. ____ a specialization in medicine concerned with the study and treatment of mental disorders
e. ____ the use of medication to treat mental disorders
f. ____ Governing offices that provide licenses to practice to health professionals
g. ____ a legal term indicating a legal defense or finding that, although a person committed a crime, he or she is not criminally responsible for the behaviour because of a mental disorder
h. ____ a movement founded on a basic respect for human dignity and the belief that humanistic care would be effective in the treatment of mental illness, that promoted improved conditions at mental hospitals

i. _____ the use of psychological procedures in the context of a relationship with a therapist to treat mental disorders

j. _____ the alternative to the experimental hypothesis; predicts that the experimental hypothesis is not true

k. _____ currently, this is a legal term referring to a person's culpability for criminal acts if he or she has a mental disorder

l. _____ another term for disorganized speech

m. _____ an approach to defining whether a condition is a mental disorder in terms of its harm to the person and whether the condition results from the inability of some mental mechanism to perform its natural function

n. _____ a specialization in psychology concerned with the application of psychological science to the assessment and treatment of mental disorders

o. _____ the values, beliefs and practices that are shared by a specific community or group of people

p. _____ the official listing of mental disorders and their diagnostic criteria published by the American Psychiatric Association and updated regularly

q. _____ a profession concerned with helping people achieve an effective level of psychosocial functioning; focuses less on a body of scientific knowledge than on a commitment to action

r. _____ the debate over whether genetic or biological factors versus environmental factors cause mental disorders or abnormal behaviour

s. _____ an old-fashioned term indicating that a person became incapacitated because of an unspecified mental disorder

t. _____ the analytic approach toward etiology combining the influences of biological, psychological, and social systems

u. _____ psychopathology based on the signs and symptoms of a mental disorder rather than on its inferred causes

v. _____ a degree including nursing in addition to additional training in mental health issues

w. _____ master's level care providers focusing on offering direct service

x. _____ professionals who teach the severely mentally ill practical daily living skills

y. _____ masters' level treatment providers with a theoretical orientation focusing on couples and family issues

Names You Should Know — Matching

The following people or legal cases have played an important role in abnormal psychology. To test your knowledge, match the following names with the descriptions of their contributions. Answers are listed at the end of the chapter.

    a. Jerome Wakefield   c. Dorothea Dix
    b. Hippocrates   d. Dr. Ewen Cameron

1. _____ an early advocate for the humane treatment of the mentally ill; promoted the creation of mental institutions for treatment

2.   ____   saw mental disorders as diseases having natural causes, like other forms of physical diseases

3.   ____   developed an experimental treatment called psychic driving, which he intended as a "brainwashing" method for eradicating bad behaviour patterns; optimistic about curing mental Illnesses

4.   ____   proposed the harmful dysfunction approach to defining mental disorder

Review of Concepts — Fill in the Blank and True/False

This section will help focus your studying by testing whether you understand the concepts presented in the text. After you have read and reviewed the material, test your comprehension and memory by filling in the following blanks or circling the right answer. Answers are listed at the end of the chapter.

1.   Case studies are particularly important in understanding mental disorders that are

_____.

2.   Case studies can prove that a certain factor is the cause of a disorder:

   true   false

3.   One limitation of case studies is that one person may not be _____

of the disorder as a whole.

4.   There are several laboratory tests available to test for the presence of certain forms

of mental disorders: **true   false**

5.   An unusual behaviour or symptom that goes away after a few days is not clinically

significant; that is, it does not indicate that a person has a disorder:

   true   false

6.   What is the problem with defining abnormal behaviour based on the individual's

experience of personal distress? _____

7.   What is the problem with defining abnormal behaviour based on statistical norms

of rarity? _____

8.   The DSM-IV defines mental disorder in terms of personal _____ or

impairment of _____ or with significantly increased risk of

suffering some form of harm, whether death, injury, or loss of freedom.

9. Why was the behaviour of the Yippie Party of the 1960's, whose members threw money off the balcony at a stock exchange, not considered to be a symptom of a mental illness? _____

10. The DSM-IV is not influenced by social or cultural forces: **true   false**

11. Why does the DSM no longer consider homosexuality to be a mental disorder?

    _____

12. What type of approach does the DSM-IV take to classifying mental disorders? **dimensional   categorical**

13. Much of our current estimates of the prevalence of mental disorder is based on the _____ study.

14. Most psychopathologists view mental disorders as being culture-free:

    true   false

15. Psychotic disorders are less influenced by culture than are nonpsychotic disorders:

    true   false

16. Epidemiological studies indicate that the following percent of people had at least one diagnosable condition sometime in their life: **6%   32%   83%**

17. People affected by severe disorders often qualify for the diagnosis of more than one disorder at the same time: **true   false**

18. The concept of disease burden combines which two factors? _____ and _____

19. Mental disorders cause 1% of all deaths but produce 47% of all _____ in economically developed countries.

20. Almost all mental disorders occur in Western countries: **true   false**

21. Scientists have come to fairly well-agreed-upon conclusions about the etiology of most mental disorders: **true   false**

22. A psychopathologist who hypothesizes that schizophrenia is caused by an infectious agent, like a virus, would be arguing for which side of the controversy:

    nature   nurture

23. Almost all patients who are being treated in psychotherapy are not treated with medication at the same time: **true**   **false**

24. Most people who have a diagnosable mental disorder receive some form of treatment for it: **true**   **false**

25. Why is it an error to conclude that when a treatment is successful in relieving a mental disorder, that treatment indicates the cause of the disorder?

    _____

    _____

26. Many ancient theories of abnormal behaviour see as its cause the disfavor of the gods or demonic possession: **true**   **false**

27. Cutting patients to make them bleed and reduce the amount of blood in the body was a form of treatment for mental illness in the 19th century   **true**   **false**

28. Urbanization was one of the reasons that_____ were built.

29. What led to the creation of the medical speciality of psychiatry? _____

    _____

30. Mental health professionals at the beginning of the nineteenth century such as William Tuke and Philip Pinel advocated _____ as a new approach to relieving mental illness.

31. Dr. Awl (A.K.A. Dr. "Cure-Awl") claimed a success rate in treating his institutionalized mental patients of: **about 30%**   **about 50%**   **100%**

32. Fever therapy involved infecting mental patients with _____ to cause a fever because symptoms sometimes disappeared in patients with a high fever.

33. What type of mental health professionals can prescribe medication?_____

    _____

34. What type of mental health professionals are trained in the use of scientific research methods?_____

35. More and more of the treatment providers for mental health services are profes-
     sionals other than physicians: **true**   **false**

Multiple Choice Questions

The following multiple choice questions will test your comprehension of the material presented in the chapter. Answers are listed at the end of the chapter.

1)   A type of formal thought disorder which has the prominent feature of severe disrup-
     tions of verbal communication.

     a. depression   c. psychosis
     b. schizophrenia   d. disorganized speech

2)   This model combines the dimensional and categorical approaches to classification.

     a. threshold model   c. diathesis-stress model
     b. scientist-practioner model   d. biopsychosocial model

3)   When literally translated, the term "psychopathology" refers to:

     a. "deterioration of the psyche"   c. "pathology of the psyche"
     b. pathology of the mind   d. "deterioration of the mind"

4)   A mental disorder is typically defined by:

     a. a person experiencing the feeling that something is wrong
     b. statistical rarity
     c. a set of characteristic features
     d. being out of contact with reality

5)   Beth shows delusional thinking and hallucinations. Bob shows hallucinations and
     formal thought disorder. According to DSM-IV:

     a. they could both be classified as schizophrenic
     b. they would be given different diagnoses
     c. they probably have different etiologies
     d. they should get different treatments

6)   All of the following are hypotheses of the etiology of abnormal behaviour EXCEPT:

     a. diathesis-stress model   c. biological reductionism
     b. biopsychosocial model   d. scientist-practitioner model

7) The approach that defines psychopathology in terms of signs and symptoms rather than inferred causes is:

   a. descriptive psychopathology
   b. influential psychopathology
   c. comparative psychopathology
   d. experiential psychopathology

8) All of the following are ways in which case studies can be useful EXCEPT:

   a. provide important insights about the nature of mental disorders
   b. allow you to draw conclusions about a disorder from a single experience
   c. aid a clinician in making hypotheses about a specific case
   d. provide a rich clinical description which can be helpful in diagnosing an individual

9) These two disorders are much more common in men than they are in women.

   a. alcoholism; antisocial personality disorder
   b. anxiety disorders; depression
   c. alcoholism; depression
   d. anxiety disorders; antisocial personality disorder

10) All of the following could be considered psychotic symptoms EXCEPT:

   a. delusions
   b. hallucinations
   c. disorganized speech
   d. depression

11) Eating disorders can be fatal if they are not properly treated because:

   a. there is a high suicide rate among people with eating disorders
   b. they affect so many vital organs of the body
   c. people with eating disorders are often unaware of the disorder and therefore are prone to developing additional disorders
   d. the majority of people with eating disorders do not view their behaviour as problematic and therefore do not seek treatment

12) Cultural forces:

   a. mostly affect people living in non-Western societies
   b. do not change
   c. only affect women
   d. affect what we perceive as abnormal

13) This is a general term that refers to a type of severe mental disorder in which the individual is considered to be out of contact with reality.

   a. threshold
   b. syndrome
   c. psychosis
   d. schizophrenia

14) _____ is to experience as _____ is to genes.

    a. nature; nurture
    b. nurture; nature

    c. quantitative; qualitative
    d. qualitative; quantitative

15) In order for a behaviour to be considered abnormal, it must include all of the following EXCEPT:

    a. present distress or painful symptoms
    b. conflicts between the individual and society that are voluntary in nature
    c. impairment in one or more important areas of functioning
    d. increased risk of suffering death, pain, disability, or an important loss of freedom

16) Which is true about the role of value judgments in the development of diagnostic systems?

    a. values can be avoided with the use of scientific methods
    b. diagnosis is completely determined by values
    c. values have no place in the attempt to define disease
    d. values are inherent in any attempt to define disease

17) The conclusion of Jane Murphy's study of the Inuit of Northwest Alaska and the Yoruba of rural, tropical Nigeria was that severe forms of mental illness:

    a. are not limited to Western cultures or developed countries
    b. do appear to be limited to Western cultures or developed countries
    c. are more prevalent in Western cultures and developed countries
    d. are more prevalent in the Inuit and Yoruba populations studied

18) Olivia grew up in a society where mourners pull out their hair, go into an emotional frenzy, and begin speaking in tongues. On a visit to Canada, she did these things in public when she heard that a relative had died. According to DSM-IV, this would be considered:

    a. not to be psychopathology, because it is part of her culture
    b. not to be psychopathology, because it caused no disruption in her social relationships
    c. to be psychopathology, because of her personal distress
    d. to be psychopathology, because it impaired her functioning

19) Which of the following is NOT considered a criterion for defining a behaviour as a form of mental illness?

    a. negative effects on the person's social functioning
    b. recognition by the person that his or her behaviour is problematic
    c. personal discomfort
    d. persistent, maladaptive behaviours

Understanding Research – Fill in the Blank

Cross-Cultural Study of Abnormal Behaviour: The text presents a detailed description of a study by Murphy in the Research Close Up. Finding the answers to these questions will help you get a good understanding of this study and why it is important. It is not necessary to memorize the answers; the process of finding them in the textbook will help you learn the material you need to know.

1.   What did the textbook mean by the term "non-Western?" _____
_____ What were the two groups of people
Murphy studied? _____ and _____. She lived
with each of them for several _____, learned their languages, and
learned how they think about problem _____.

2.   Both cultures recognize certain forms of "crazy" behaviour, including aberrant
beliefs, feelings, and actions, hearing _____, _____ at
strange times, talking in ways that don't make _____: which are like
what diagnosis? _____. The specific _____ of hallu-
cinations and delusions varies from one culture to the next, but the underlying
_____appear to be the same. Both groups saw "crazy
behaviour" as being different from the behaviours of the _____, who
also acted strangely at times when doing their job. "When the shaman is
healing, he is out of his mind, but he is not_____."

3.   Both groups believe that mental illness originates in _____.
Their attitudes toward "crazy" people were neither _____ nor
_____. The World _____ Organization studied
schizophrenia in _____ countries and found about the same
_____of the disorder in all the countries.

The Null Hypothesis and the Burden of Proof: The text discusses this research issue in the Research Methods sections. Finding the answers to these questions will help you get a good understanding of these issues.

4.   What is the rule that scientists agree upon for making and testing any new hypothesis?

_____

_____

The two hypotheses set up in any research study are the _____ hypothesis and the _____hypothesis. This rule is similar to the legal saying: _____. These are both _____ principals designed to protect the field from _____ assertions. Scientists feel that _____ "scientific evidence" is more dangerous than _____ knowledge.

5. Lists three examples of treatment that were used in the past on many thousands of patients without established effectiveness: _____ , _____, and _____. What are some of the modern treatments that should be shown effective before their use: _____. Scientists do not prove the Null Hypothesis; they only fail to _____ it.

Brief Essay

As a final exercise, write out answers to the following brief essay questions. Then compare your answers with the material presented in the text.

After you have answered these questions, review the "critical thinking" questions that are presented at the end of the text chapter. Answering these questions will help you integrate important issues and themes that have been featured throughout the chapter.

1. Briefly describe the criteria that need to be present in order for a behaviour to be considered "abnormal." Why is it important to have criteria in order to define a behaviour as "abnormal?"

2. Compare and contrast the various approaches presented in this chapter that attempt to explain the etiology of abnormal behaviour. What are the strengths and weaknesses of these models?

3. Choose one of the four case studies presented in this chapter and briefly describe the importance of the case in learning about the disorder. In what ways is this case similar to the other three cases? What are some issues that are unique to this case? What can be learned from studying case studies?

ANSWER KEY

Key Terms – Matching #1

1. e	8. r	15. f
2. a	9. d	16. k
3. o	10. c	17. b
4. h	11. g	18. m
5. i	12. s	19. p
6. l	13. n	
7. q	14. j	

Key Terms — Matching #2

a. 7	g. 3	m. 9	s. 4	y. 23
b. 18	h. 16	n. 20	t. 12	
c. 6	i. 14	o. 15	u. 5	
d. 17	j. 19	p. 10	v. 24	
e. 13	k. 2	q. 21	w. 22	
f. 8	l. 1	r. 11	x. 25	

Multiple Choice

1. d	6. d	11. b	16. d
2. a	7. a	12. d	17. a
3. b	8. b	13. c	18. b
4. c	9. a	14. b	19. b
5. a	10. d	15. b	

Names You Should Know

1. c
2. b
3. d
4. a

Review of Concepts

1. rare
2. **false**
3. representative
4. **false**
5. true
6. they may not have insight
7. something rare is not necessarily bad
8. distress; functioning
9. it was voluntary and was a political gesture
10. **false**
11. political pressure from gay rights activists
12. categorical
13. Cross-National Collaborative Study
14. **false**
15. true
16. 32%
17. true
18. mortality and disability
19. disability
20. **false**
21. **false**
22. nature
23. **false**
24. **false**
25. it's a logical error, like thinking a lack of aspirin causes headaches

26. true
27. true
28. lunatic asylums
29. creation of institutions to treat mental patients
30. respect for human dignity and humanistic care

31. 100%
32. malaria
33. psychiatrists
34. Ph.D. clinical psychologists
35. true

Understanding Research

1. People living in non-industrialized or undeveloped cultures or countries, or other than the U.S., Canada, and Europe; Inuits and the Yoruba; months; behaviours

2. voices; laughing; sense; schizophrenia; content; processes; shamans; crazy

3. magic; positive; negative; Health; 9; frequency

4. The scientist who makes a new prediction must prove it to be true; experimental; null; innocent until proven guilty; conservative; false; undetected

5. lobotomies; fever therapy; coma therapy; institutionalization, medication, and psychotherapy; reject

CHAPTER 2
CAUSES OF ABNORMAL BEHAVIOUR:
FROM PARADIGMS TO SYSTEMS

Chapter Outline

I. Overview

II. Brief Historical Perspective: 20th Century Paradigms
    A. General Paresis and the Biological Paradigm
    B. Freud and the Psychodynamic Paradigm
    C. Psychology, Learning, and the Cognitive Behavioural Paradigm
    D. Free Will and the Humanistic Paradigm
    E. The Problem with Paradigms

III. Systems Theory
    A. Holism
       1. Reductionism
       2. Levels of Analysis
    B. Causality: Multiple Factors and Multiple Pathways
       1. The Diathesis-Stress Model
       2. Equifinality and Multifinality
    C. Reciprocal Causality
    D. Development

IV. Biological Factors
    A. The Neuron and Neurotransmitters
       1. Neurotransmitters and the Aetiology of Psychopathology
    B. Major Brain Structures
       1. Cerebral Hemispheres
       2. Major Brain Structures and the Aetiology of Psychopathology
    C. Psychophysiology
       1. Endocrine System
       2. Autonomic Nervous System
       3. Psychophysiology and the Aetiology of Psychopathology
    D. Behaviour Genetics
       1. Some Basic Principles of Genetics
       2. Twin Studies
    E. Adoption Studies
       1. Family Incidence Studies
    F. Misinterpreting Behaviour Genetics Findings
       1. Genetics and the Aetiology of Psychopathology

V. Psychological Factors
    A. Motivation, Emotion, and Temperament
        1. Hierarchy of Need
        2. Attachment Theory
        3. Dominance Relations
        4. Emotions and Emotional Systems
        5. Temperament
        6. Motivation, Emotion, Temperament, and the Aetiology of Psychopathology
    B. Learning and Cognition
        1. Modelling
        2. Social Cognition
        3. Learning, Distorted Cognition, and the Aetiology of Psychopathology
    C. The Sense of Self
        1. Self Systems and the Aetiology of Psychopathology
    D. Stages of Development
        1. Development and the Aetiology of Psychopathology

VI. Social Factors
    A. Relationships and Psychopathology
        1. Marital Status and Psychopathology
        2. Social Relationships
    B. Gender and Gender Roles
    C. Race and Poverty
    D. Societal Values

Learning Objectives

After reviewing the material presented in this chapter, you should be able to:

1. Define the biopsychosocial approach and explain how it is a systems approach.

2. Name some of the major breakthroughs that led to modern scientific abnormal psychology: a) discovery of the biological origins of general paresis, b) Freud's talking cure with hysterical patients, and c) emergence of scientific academic psychology (Wundt, Pavlov, Skinner, Watson, etc.).

3. Distinguish holism from reductionism.

4. Understand how systems theory replaces the 4 paradigms of the 20th century.

5. Understand various aspects about aetiology: pathology can be caused by multiple factors/pathways; correlation does not mean cause; equifinality means that a disorder may have many different causes for different incidences of the disease; diathesis-stress models imply both predisposition and a stressful event may precipitate a disorder.

6. Describe the basic functions of the hindbrain, midbrain, and forebrain.

7. Distinguish structural from psychophysiological problems.

8. Separate central from peripheral nervous systems; voluntary vs. autonomic nervous systems; sympathetic vs. parasympathetic nervous system.

9. Know the basic research design used for twin studies, adoption studies, and family incidence studies.

10. Define temperament and explain its significance in the aetiology of psychopathology.

11. Describe some ways in which modeling, social cognition, and sense of self may affect abnormal behaviour.

12. Understand that the following social factors are generally correlated (not causative) with psychopathology: relationship difficulties, gender, race, and poverty.

Key Terms — Matching #1

The following terms related to abnormal psychology are important to know. To test your knowledge, match the following terms with their definitions. Answers are listed at the end of the chapter.

a.	Paradigm	m.	Reality principle
b.	Multifactional causes	n.	Superego
c.	Biological paradigm	o.	Neurotic anxiety
d.	General paresis	p.	Defence mechanisms
e.	Syphilis	q.	Projection
f.	Psychoanalytic theory	r.	Psychosexual development
g.	Hysteria	s.	Oedipal conflict
h.	Conversion disorder	t.	Electra complex
i.	Libido	u.	Unconscious
j.	Pleasure principle	v.	Moral anxiety
k.	Id	w.	Cognitive behavioural paradigm
l.	Ego	x.	Psychodynamic paradigm

1. _____ an elaborate theory of personality proposed by Freud that focuses on basic biological and psychological drives.

2. _____ a set of assumptions about the substance of a theory and the scientific method used to test the theory

3. _____ unconscious processes that reduce conscious anxiety by distorting conflictual memories, emotions, and impulses

4. _____ the mode of operation for the ego, where the need to gratify impulses is balanced with demands of reality

5. ____ Freud's concept that a stage boys go through involves having sexual impulses toward their mothers and aggressive impulses toward their fathers, which is resolved by identifying with their fathers

6. ____ a psychoanalytic diagnostic category involving the conversion of psychological conflicts into physical symptoms

7. ____ Freud's theory of development

8. ____ a sexually transmitted disease caused by bacteria, the end stage of which includes psychiatric symptoms; treatable with antibiotics

9. ____ a Freudian term for the part of personality which serves as the conscience, containing societal standards of behaviour

10. ____ the modern diagnostic category for hysteria

11. ____ a Freudian term for the part of personality which is the source of basic drives and motivations, including sexual and aggressive impulses

12. ____ the aetiology of a disorder results from a combination of biological, psychological, and social factors

13. ____ produced by conflict between the id and the ego

14. ____ Freud's concept that a stage girls go through involves yearning for a penis, which they feel they must have lost

15. ____ focuses on biological causation

16. ____ a defence mechanism where the person perceives his or her own forbidden unconscious impulses as a characteristic of another person

17. ____ a Freudian term for sexual or life energy

18. ____ the mode of operation for the id, where impulses seek immediate gratification

19. ____ a disorder with delusions of grandeur, dementia, and progressive paralysis; progressively worsens, ending in death; caused by untreated syphilis

20. ____ a Freudian term for the part of personality which deals with the realities of the world

21. ____ mental processes or contents outside of a person's awareness, largely unavailable to the person

22. ____ produced by conflict between the ego and superego

23. ____ views abnormal behaviour as caused by unconscious conflicts arising out of early childhood experiences

24. ____ assert that behaviour is learned and examines the processes underlying learning

Key Terms — Matching #2

The following terms related to abnormal psychology are important to know. To test your knowledge, match the following terms with their definitions. Answers are listed at the end of the chapter.

1. Introspection
2. Classical conditioning
3. Unconditioned stimulus
4. Unconditioned response
5. Conditioned stimulus
6. Conditioned response
7. Extinction
8. Operant conditioning
9. Positive reinforcement
10. Negative reinforcement

11. Punishment
12. Response cost
13. Behaviourism
14. Humanistic psychology
15. Determinism
16. Free will
17. Systems theory
18. Holism
19. Reductionism
20. Risk factors
21. Molecular
22. Molar
23. Levels of analysis
24. Correlational study
25. Correlational coefficent

a. _____ a neutral stimulus that, when repeatedly paired with a stimulus that elicits an automatic reaction, comes to produce that reaction itself
b. _____ the idea that human behaviour is determined by a person's choice and free will.
c. _____ the statistic for measuring how strongly two factors are related; it ranges between -1.0 and +1.0
d. _____ when the onset of a stimulus increases the frequency of a behaviour
e. _____ the use of different perspectives, subsystems, or "lenses" to conceptualize causal factors
f. _____ when the removal of a stimulus decreases the frequency of behaviour
g. _____ focus on inner experiences
h. _____ events or circumstances that are correlated with an increased likelihood of a disorder
i. _____ a paradigm that emphasizes interdependence, cybernetics, and holism
j. _____ Pavlov's form of learning through association of paired stimuli
k. _____ a research design where the relation between two factors is studied
l. _____ when the cessation of a stimulus increases the frequency of a behaviour
m. _____ a stimulus that elicits an automatic reaction
n. _____ the assumption that human behaviour is caused by predictable and potentially knowable internal and/or external events
o. _____ an automatic reaction to an event
p. _____ the most general
q. _____ the belief within psychology that observable behaviours are the only appropriate focus of psychological study
r. _____ a learning theory asserting that behaviour is a function of its consequences; that behaviour increases if it is rewarded and decreases if it is punished
s. _____ the gradual elimination of a response when learning conditions change
t. _____ the idea that the whole is more than the sum of its parts
u. _____ the most reductionistic
v. _____ the perspective that the whole is the sum of its parts, and that the task for science is to divide the world into smaller and smaller components
w. _____ when the introduction of a stimulus decreases the frequency of a behaviour
x. _____ a paradigm of abnormal behaviour that rejects determinism and argues that human behaviour is the product of free will
y. _____ a response that is elicited by a conditioned stimulus

Key Terms — Matching #3

The following terms related to abnormal psychology are important to know. To test your knowledge, match the following terms with their definitions. Answers are listed at the end of the chapter.

a. Positive correlations
b. Negative correlations
c. Third-variable
d. Diathesis-stress model
e. Equifinality
f. Reciprocal causality
g. Linear causality
h. Cybernetics
i. Homeostasis
j. Developmental psychopathology
k. Developmental norms
l. Premorbid history
m. Reverse causality

n. Prognosis
o. Anatomy
p. Physiology
q. Neuroanatomy
r. Neurophysiology
s. Neurons
t. Soma
u. Dendrites
v. Axon
w. Axon Terminal
x. Synapse
y. Neurotransmitters
z. Multifinality

1. ____ a communication and control process that uses feedback loops in order to adjust progress toward a goal
2. ____ the study of brain structures
3. ____ a pattern of behaviour that precedes the onset of the disorder
4. ____ trunk of the neuron that transmits messages toward other cells
5. ____ the idea that causality is bidirectional
6. ____ cell body
7. ____ predictions about the future course of a disorder
8. ____ the same psychological disorder may have different causes
9. ____ the study of biological structures
10. ____ an approach to abnormal psychology that emphasizes the importance of age-graded averages and determining what constitutes abnormal behaviour
11. ____ the study of biological functions
12. ____ the end of the axon where messages are sent out to other neurons
13. ____ as one factor goes up, the other factor goes down
14. ____ age-graded averages
15. ____ as one factor goes up, the other factor goes up
16. ____ causation operates in one direction only
17. ____ branching cell structures that receive messages from other cells
18. ____ the possibility that causation could be operating in the opposite direction; Y could be causing X instead of X causing Y
19. ____ the tendency to maintain a steady state
20. ____ the study of brain functions
21. ____ a small gap between neurons that is filled with fluid

22. _____ a correlation between two variables could be explained by their joint relation with some unmeasured factor
23. _____ nerve cells
24. _____ the same event can lead to different outcomes
25. _____ chemical substances released into the synapse that carry signals from one neuron to another
26. _____ a view of the aetiology of a disorder that assumes it is produced by an interaction between a predisposition and a precipitating event

Key Terms – Matching #4

The following terms related to abnormal psychology are important to know. To test your knowledge, match the following terms with their definitions. Answers are listed at the end of the chapter.

1. Receptors	13. Limbic system
2. Reuptake	14. Thalamus
3. Neuromodulators	15. Hypothalamus
4. Vesicles	16. Cerebral hemispheres
5. Dualism	17. Lateralized
6. Hindbrain	18. Corpus callosum
7. Medulla	19. Ventricles
8. Pons	20. Cerebral cortex
9. Cerebellum	21. Frontal lobe
10. Midbrain	22. Parietal lobe
11. Reticular activating system	23. Temporal lobe
12. Forebrain	24. Occipital lobe

a. _____ a brain grouping including the medulla, pons, and cerebellum
b. _____ regulates emotion and basic learning processes
c. _____ sites on the dendrites or soma of a neuron that are sensitive to certain neurotransmitters
d. _____ the uneven surface of the brain just underneath the skull which controls and integrates sophisticated memory, sensory, and motor functions
e. _____ receives and integrates sensory information and plays a role in spatial reasoning
f. _____ controls bodily functions which sustain life, like heart rate and respiration
g. _____ the process of recapturing some neurotransmitters from the synapse before they reach the receptors of another neuron
h. _____ receives and integrates sensory information from the sense organs and from higher brain structures
i. _____ four connected chambers in the brain filled with cerebrospinal fluid
j. _____ each cerebral hemisphere serves a specialized role in brain function; the left hemisphere is involved in language and the right in spatial relations

k.   ____   regulates stages of sleep
l.   ____   connects the two cerebral hemispheres, and coordinates their different
               functions
m.   ____   helps coordinate physical movement
n.   ____   processes sound and smell, regulates emotions, and is involved in learning,
               memory, and language
o.   ____   controls a number of complex functions like reasoning, planning, emotion,
               speech, and movement
p.   ____   the view that mind and body are separable
q.   ____   regulates sleep and waking
r.   ____   a brain grouping which evolved last and is the location of most sensory,
               emotional, and cognitive processes
s.   ____   the two major structures of the forebrain and the site of most sensory, emo-
               tional, and cognitive processes
t.   ____   chemicals that may be released from neurons or endocrine glands which
               influence communications of many neurons by affecting the functioning of
               neurotransmitters
u.   ____   a brain grouping which controls some motor activities, especially fighting
               and sex, and includes part of the reticular activating system
v.   ____   receives and interprets visual information
w.   ____   controls basic biological urges such as eating, drinking, and sex
x.   ____   structures which contain neurotransmitters

Key Terms — Matching #5

The following terms related to abnormal psychology are important to know. To test your
knowledge, match the following terms with their definitions. Answers are listed at the
end of the chapter.

a.	Psychophysiology	n.	Genotype
b.	Endocrine system	o.	Phenotype
c.	Hormones	p.	Alleles
d.	Hyperthyroidism/Graves' disease	q.	Locus
e.	Central nervous system	r.	Polygenic
f.	Peripheral nervous system	s.	Monozygotic (MZ)
g.	Somatic nervous system	t.	Dizygotic (DZ)
h.	Autonomic nervous system	u.	Concordance
i.	Sympathetic nervous system	v.	Shared environment
j.	Parasympathetic nervous system	w.	Nonshared environment
k.	Genes	x.	Probands
l.	Chromosomes	y.	Individual differences
m.	Behaviour genetics	z.	Species-typical characteristics

1. ____ the study of changes in the functioning of the body that result from psychological experiences
2. ____ an individual's actual genetic structure
3. ____ fraternal twins produced from separate fertilized eggs; the twins are as genetically related as nontwin siblings
4. ____ the voluntary nervous system that governs muscular control
5. ____ chainlike structures in the nucleus of all cells
6. ____ the component of the family environment that offers the same or very similar experiences to all siblings
7. ____ a division of the human nervous system including all connections to the body's muscles, sensory systems, and organs
8. ____ the component of the family and outside of the family environment that is unique to that sibling
9. ____ a specific location on a chromosome
10. ____ a division of the human nervous system including the brain and spinal cord
11. ____ characteristics all people have in common as part of human nature
12. ____ units of DNA, located on the chromosomes, that carry information about heredity
13. ____ caused by more than one gene
14. ____ chemical substances that affect the functioning of distant body systems
15. ____ the study of genetic influences on the evolution and development of normal and abnormal behaviour
16. ____ a collection of glands located throughout the body that produce psychophysiological responses by releasing hormones into the bloodstream
17. ____ the involuntary nervous system that regulates body organs
18. ____ identical twins produced from a single fertilized egg; the twins have identical genotypes
19. ____ the expression of a given genotype
20. ____ agreement; when twin pairs either both have a disorder or both are free of the disorder
21. ____ alternate forms of a genetic trait
22. ____ how people are different from one another
23. ____ a disease where the thyroid gland secretes too much of the hormone thyroxin, causing restlessness, agitation, and anxiety
24. ____ a division of the autonomic nervous system that controls the slowing of arousal and energy conservation
25. ____ index cases; people who have a disorder and then their relatives are examined to see if they also have the disorder
26. ____ a division of the autonomic nervous system that is associated with increased arousal and expenditure of energy

Key Terms — Matching #6

The following terms related to abnormal psychology are important to know. To test your knowledge, match the following terms with their definitions. Answers are listed at the end of the chapter.

1. Hierarchy of needs	11. Agreeableness
2. Attachment theory	12. Conscientiousness
3. Ethology	13. Anxious attachments
4. Imprinting	14. Goodness of fit
5. Dominance	15. Modelling
6. Emotions	16. Identification
7. Temperament	17. Social cognition
8. Neuroticism	18. Attributions
9. Extraversion	19. Learned helplessness theory
10. Openness to experience	20. Cognitive errors

a. _____ internal feeling states

b. _____ a personality dimension of active and talkative vs. passive and reserved

c. _____ a personality dimension of trusting and kind vs. hostile and selfish

d. _____ learning through imitation of others

e. _____ the study of animal behaviour

f. _____ an ordering of human motivations according to priority by Maslow

g. _____ the study of how humans process information about themselves and others

h. _____ the theory that infants form special and selective bonds with their care-givers early in life

i. _____ uncertain or ambivalent parent-child relationships resulting from inconsistent and unresponsive parenting particularly in the first year of life

j. _____ may be related to depression; wrongly attributing negative events to internal, global, and stable causes

k. _____ a personality dimension of nervous and moody vs. calm and pleasant

l. _____ the match between children's temperaments and their environment

m. _____ automatic and distorted perceptions of reality; negative ones may be linked to depression

n. _____ a process where children not only imitate a model but want to be like it and adopt its values

o. _____ the hierarchical ordering of a social group into more and less powerful members

p. _____ an inflexible process of forming selective bonds in the first hours of life which occurs in some species

q. _____ a personality dimension of imaginative and curious vs. shallow and imperceptive

r. _____ people's beliefs about cause-effect relationships

s. _____ characteristic styles of relating to the world that are very stable

t. _____ a personality dimension of organized and reliable vs. careless and negligent

Key Terms — Matching #7

The following terms related to abnormal psychology are important to know. To test your knowledge, match the following terms with their definitions. Answers are listed at the end of the chapter.

a.	Identity	k.	Fixation
b.	Role identities	l.	Regression
c.	Self-schema	m.	Social roles
d.	Irrational beliefs	n.	Labelling theory
e.	Self-Control	o.	Self-fulfilling prophesy
f.	Socialization	p.	Social support
g.	Self-concept	q.	Gender roles
h.	Self-efficacy	r.	Relational
i.	Developmental stage	s.	Instrumental
j.	Developmental transition	t.	Androgyny

1. ____ the belief that one can achieve desired goals
2. ____ a return to an earlier stage or style of coping or behaving
3. ____ internal rules for guiding appropriate behaviour
4. ____ abnormal behaviour is created by social expectations or roles
5. ____ oriented toward others
6. ____ styles of behaving according to the expectations of the social situation
7. ____ possessing both female and male gender-role characteristics
8. ____ various senses of self which correspond with life roles
9. ____ the emotional and practical assistance received from others
10. ____ definition of self
11. ____ cognitive conceptualizations about oneself
12. ____ impossible absolute standards
13. ____ when psychological development is arrested at a particular stage
14. ____ roles associated with social expectations about gendered behaviour
15. ____ people's actions conforming to the expectations created by a label given to them
16. ____ the process where parents, teachers, and peers use discipline, praise, and example to teach children prosocial behaviour and set limits on antisocial behaviour
17. ____ feelings about one's worthiness and capability
18. ____ the idea that stressful and important changes occur during times of rapid biological, psychological, or social development
19. ____ oriented toward action and achievement
20. ____ a period of continuous and slow change

Names You Should Know — Matching

The following people have played an important role in research and theory of anxiety disorders. To test your knowledge, match the following names with the descriptions of their contributions to the study of abnormal psychology. Answers are listed at the end of the chapter.

a. Sigmund Freud
b. B. F. Skinner
c. Rene Descartes
d. John Bowlby
e. Wilhelm Wundt

f. John B. Watson
g. Gregor Mendel
h. Ivan Pavlov
i. Thomas Kuhn
j. Abraham Maslow

1. ____ attempted to balance religious teachings with emerging scientific reasoning by proposing dualism
2. ____ founded behaviourism and applied learning theory to the study of abnormal behaviour
3. ____ developed attachment theory, based in part on ethology
4. ____ developed psychoanalytic theory; focused on the importance of early child-hood experiences and unconscious conflicts
5. ____ conducted a series of studies on classical conditioning
6. ____ applied the idea of paradigm to the historical study of science
7. ____ discovered genetic inheritance; made the distinction between genotypes and phenotypes
8. ____ a humanistic psychologist who explored motivation
9. ____ one of the first experimental psychologist; pioneered the scientific study of psychological phenomena
10. ____ conducted a series of studies on operant conditioning

Review of Concepts — fill in the blank and True/False

This section will help focus your studying by testing whether you understand the concepts presented in the text. After you have read and reviewed the material, test your comprehension and memory by filling in the following blanks or circling the right answer. Answers are listed at the end of the chapter.

1. It is likely that continuing research will answer the "nature-nurture" debate by

   demonstrating on a disorder-by-disorder basis what the cause of each disorder is:

   true   false

2. What three major events encouraged advances in the scientific understanding of

   the aetiology of psychopathology in the nineteenth and twentieth centuries?

_____, _____ , and

_____.

3. The development of a _____ for general paresis inspired a search for its cause, which took 100 years of investigation.

4. General paresis was eliminated with the advent of _____.

5. The elimination of general paresis encouraged researchers to adopt what paradigm in their research on aetiology of mental disorders? _____

6. What theorist opposed the biological paradigm for mental disorders? _____

7. Freud developed his theories largely on the basis of _____ rather than scientific research.

8. What approach did Wundt use in studying psychological phenomena, which was his greatest contribution to psychology? _____

9. Cognitive behaviourists are primarily concerned with the _____ of mental disorders rather than understanding their causes.

10. _____ psychology was a reaction against biomedical, psychoanalytic, and behavioural theories of abnormal behaviour.

11. Humanistic psychologists tend to blame dysfunctional, abnormal, or aggressive behaviour on: **the individual   society**

12. What are the four paradigms the authors of your text focus on in explaining mental disorders? _____ , _____, _____, and _____

13. The textbook example of the Martian scientists trying to figure out what causes automobiles to move points out the importance of the _____ that a research approach uses.

14. A predisposition toward developing a disorder is called a: **stress   diathesis**

15. A thermostat is a good example which systems theory concept? _____

16. The density and sensitivity of _____ on neurons has been implicated in some types of abnormal behaviour.

17. All psychological experience has a representation in the biochemistry of the

    _____.

18. A _____ is caused by blood vessels in the brain rupturing and
    cutting off the supply of oxygen to parts of the brain, thereby killing surrounding
    brain tissue.

19. Psychophysiological overarousal or underarousal has been hypothesized to be
    responsible for excessive anxiety; while psychophysiological overarousal or under-
    arousal has been linked with antisocial behaviour.

20. The simple mode of dominant/recessive inheritance has been linked with forms of
    which of the following kinds of abnormal behaviour?

    schizophrenia   mental retardation   depression

21. The genetic contributions to most disorders are hypothesized to be caused by:

    a single gene   multiple genes

22. If a disorder is purely genetic, the concordance for MZ twins would be _____%
    and the concordance for DZ twins would be _____%.

23. If the concordance rates for MZ and DZ twins are the same, then what type of
    factors are responsible for the disorder?   **genetic   environmental**

24. Family incidence studies ask whether diseases _____.

25. If a disorder is shown to be genetic, then nothing can change it: **true   false**

26. According to attachment theorists, displays of distress by human infants serve to
    keep caregivers in _____, making infants more likely to survive.

27. Emotions are often experienced grouped in a constellation or system rather than
    alone: **true   false**

28. The most effective parents are those who provide both high levels of _____
    and _____

29. Two prominent stage theories are those proposed by which theorists?
    _____ and _____

30. There is a correlation between marital status of parents and emotional _____ of children.

31. A close relationship with an adult outside the family can protect children from the effects of troubled family circumstances: **true**   **false**

32. Some theorists have suggested that _____ are responsible for the much higher rates of depression among women.

33. Children from poorer neighbourhoods are more likely to be witnesses or victims of _____ in their own neighbourhoods relative to children in wealthier neighbourhoods.

Multiple Choice Questions

The following multiple choice questions will test your comprehension of the material presented in the chapter. Answers are listed at the end of the chapter.

1) Which of the following is a model that views psychopathology as resulting from physical factors that form a predisposition combined with a threatening or challenging experience?

   a. medical model
   b. diathesis-stress model
   c. threshold model
   d. biopsychosocial model

2) The assumption that biological explanations are more useful than psychological explanations because they deal with smaller units is called:

   a. biological perspective
   b. genetic predisposition
   c. biological reductionism
   d. medical model

3) Which regulates the functions of various organs such as the heart and stomach?

   a. somatic nervous system
   b. autonomic nervous system
   c. sympathetic nervous system
   d. parasympathetic nervous system

4) According to Freud, this is the part of the personality that attempts to fulfill id impulses while at the same time dealing with the realities of the world.

   a. ego
   b. id
   c. superego
   d. libido

5) All of the following are methods of learning EXCEPT:

a. classical conditioning   c. introjection
b. operant conditioning   d. modelling

6) Leading developmental theory speculates that children whose parents are
_____ and _____are better adjusted than those whose parents
are inadequate on one or both of these dimensions.

a. loving; firm in their discipline
b. authoritative; hold high expectations of their child
c. demanding; promote individuality
d. congenial; encourage separation and independence

7) Freud was trained by this neurologist who successfully used hypnosis to treat what
used to be called hysteria.

a. B. F. Skinner   c. Fritz Perls
b. Albert Bandura   d. Jean Charcot

8) While watching her daughter play kickball in the street of their neighborhood, Mrs.
Jones sees her daughter fatally being hit by a car. Soon thereafter, Mrs. Jones
loses her vision. After visits to numerous doctors, there is no known organic impairment to cause the blindness.   What would her diagnosis be?

a. depression   c. hysteria
b. conversion disorder   d. hypochondriasis

9) Which of the following could be considered an uncertain or ambivalent parent-child
relationship that is a consequence of inconsistent and unresponsive parenting, particularly during the first year of life?

a. anxious attachment   c. oppositional attachment
b. neurotic attachment   d. apathetic attachment

10) All of the following are associated with the humanistic approach EXCEPT:

a. Carl Rogers   c. Fritz Perls
b. B.F. Skinner   d. Abraham Maslow

11) In the famous experiments on which classical conditioning was based, the bell
served as the _____ and the meat powder was the _____.

a. conditioned response; unconditioned response
b. unconditioned response; conditioned response
c. conditioned stimulus; unconditioned stimulus
d. unconditioned stimulus; conditioned stimulus

12) The enigma written by Lord Byron and presented in this chapter illustrates that:

   a. paradigms are unscientific and should not be used in evaluating situations
   b. the hidden meanings in life are sometimes difficult to comprehend, however the use of a paradigm can aid in this process
   c. we should use our paradigm to reveal the meaning from certain situations
   d. assumptions made by a paradigm can at times act as blinders and lead an investigator to overlook what otherwise might be obvious

13) Mike's mother took away his privilege to use the computer for two days because he hit his sister. This is an example of:

   a. punishment
   b. response cost
   c. extinction
   d. negative reinforcement

14) Systems theory has roots in all of the following EXCEPT:

   a. biology
   b. engineering
   c. philosophy
   d. all of the above

15) _____ are chainlike structures that are found in the nucleus of cells.

   a. neurotransmitters
   b. genes
   c. chromosomes
   d. lobes

16) Which is a pattern of behaviour that precedes the onset of the disorder?

   a. prognosis
   b. premorbid history
   c. determinism
   d. self-fulfilling prophesy

17) Advances in the scientific understanding of the aetiology of psychopathology did not appear until the nineteenth and early twentieth centuries when all of the following major events occurred EXCEPT:

   a. the number of people diagnosed with some form of psychopathology rapidly increased
   b. the cause of general paresis was discovered
   c. the emergence of Sigmund Freud
   d. the creation of a new academic discipline called psychology

18) According to Freud's theory of psychosexual development, boys harbouring forbidden sexual desires for their mothers is called (a/an):

   a. defence mechanism
   b. neurotic anxiety
   c. Electra complex
   d. Oedipal conflict

19) According to the "Big Five" bipolar dimensions of personality, this domain is characterized by trusting and kind versus hostile and selfish.

a. conscientiousness
b. agreeableness
c. neuroticism
d. extraversion

20) According to the psychodynamic paradigm, the cause of abnormality is:

a. early childhood experiences
b. social learning
c. frustrations of society
d. genes, infection, or other physical damage

21) The cornerstone of humanistic psychology, _____ is the assumption that human behaviour is not determined but is a product of how people choose to act.

a. holism
b. self-fulfilling prophesy
c. individuation
d. free will

22) Which of the following is a communication and control process that uses feedback loops to adjust progress toward a goal?

a. homeostasis
b. neuromodulators
c. cybernetics
d. neurotransmitters

23) This nervous system is responsible for controlling activities associated with increased arousal and energy expenditure.

a. sympathetic nervous system
b. parasympathetic nervous system
c. autonomic nervous system
d. somatic nervous system

24) Freud can be credited with all of the following EXCEPT:

a. offering specific, empirically-derived hypotheses about his theory
b. calling attention to unconscious processes
c. formulating a stage theory of child development
d. identifying numerous intrapsychic defences

25) Which of the following are characteristic ways of behaving according to the expectations of the social situation?

a. prescribed roles
b. social roles
c. gender roles
d. transitional roles

26) All of the following are true from a systems perspective regarding the aetiology of psychopathology EXCEPT:

   a. there may be biopsychosocial contributions to psychopathology, but clear hypotheses must still be supported by empirical evidence
   b. social domains of behaviour are the most significant contribution to the causes of abnormal behaviour
   c. different types of abnormal behaviour have very different causes
   d. causes of almost all forms of abnormal behaviour are unknown at present

27) According to the behavioural paradigm, the inborn human nature is:

   a. aggressive
   b. basically good
   c. basically selfish, but having some altruism
   d. neutral, like a blank slate

28) Which of the following is a defence mechanism that includes the insistence that an experience, memory, or internal need did not occur or does not exist?

   a. sublimation   c. denial
   b. reaction formation   d. repression

29) This occurs when a conditioned stimulus is no longer presented together with an unconditioned stimulus.

   a. extinction   c. negative reinforcement
   b. punishment   d. response cost

30) A _____ is an individual's actual genetic structure.

   a. locus   c. negative reinforcement
   b. phenotype   d. response cost

31) This theory suggests that depression is caused by wrongly attributing bad events to internal, global, and stable causes.

   a. labelling theory   c. modelling theory
   b. learned helplessness theory d. social cognition theory

32) The concept that on particular event can lead to different outcomes is known as:

   a. reciprocal causality   c. linear causality
   b. equifinality   d. multifinality

Understanding Research — Fill in the Blank

Marriage and Mental Health: The text presents a detailed description of a study by Robins and Regier on the ECA in the Research Close-Up. Finding the answers to these questions will help you get a good understanding of this study and why it is important. It is not necessary to memorize the answers; the process of finding them in the textbook will help you learn the material you need to know.

1. A factor commonly found to be correlated with psychological well-being is

    _____. This study, the _____study, involved interviewing

    _____ of people. There were consistent correlations between marriage

    and _____health. Of people still in their first marriage, _____% were diag-

    nosed with depression in the past year; of people who were never married, the rate

    was ____%; among those divorced once the rate was _____%; among those

    divorced more than once the rate was _____%.

2. What other diagnostic category was found to be correlated with marital status?

    _____ What percentage of people in their first marriage had ever had

    this diagnosis? _____%. What percentage of people never married?_____%

    What percentage of people divorced once? _____% What percentage of people

    divorced more than once? _____% Another disorder that was correlated was

    _____. Marital status was correlated with virtually _____

    psychological disorder that was diagnosed in this study.

3. One explanation for these findings is that not being married_____

    mental disorders, because having a spouse may provide emotional support, and

    divorce and _____and loss of support may increase susceptibility to

    disorders. However, emotional problems may _____marital status.

    Psychologically disturbed people may have more trouble _____and forming

    relationships, and may have shakier marriages. This explanation is called

    _____. Another explanation is the _____ interpreta-

    tion, which states that another factor may cause a _____ correlation

    between marital status and abnormal behaviour. One possible factor to consider is

    _____.

4. These different explanations result in very different implications for _____ of mental disorders and social _____. What should be done if the third variable hypothesis is correct? _____ What do most researchers conclude about the correlation between marriage and mental health? It remains after controlling for _____variables; for disorders like schizophrenia, marital status is a reaction to, not a cause of, the _____ problem; and marital status does have causal impact on disorders like _____.

The Correlational Study: The text discusses this type of research in the Research Methods section. Finding the answers to these questions will help you get a good understanding of these issues.

5. In a correlational study, the relation between two _____ is studied systematically. The statistic that measures how strongly two factors are related is the correlation _____, which ranges between _____. If the correlation is positive, that means that as one factor goes up, the other factor goes _____. What are two examples of positive correlations given? _____ If the correlation is negative, that means that as one factor goes up, the other factor goes _____. One note of caution is that correlation does not mean_____.

6. What are the two alternative explanations besides one factor causing the other? _____ and _____ What does spurious mean? _____

    _____

Canadian Focus: The text presents a brief history of a failed attempt by the Canadian government during the 1800s to implement a series of reforms to encourage First Nations people to assimilate into European culture.

7. At that time, the Canadian government failed to understand the _____ of First Nations cultures, and erroneously assumed that European culture was _____. Consequently, First Nations _____ were banned and

children were _____. The goal of the programme was to get First Nations children while they were young and place them in _____ where they learned to _____. However, the main goal was to remove them from _____. Although the original goal of the programme was to help First Nations people _____ into European culture, the result was that First Nations families _____ and First Nations people were made to feel that they were _____ . Many school children were victims of _____ as well.

Brief Essay

As a final exercise, write out answers to the following brief essay questions. Then compare your answers with the material presented in the text.

After you have answered these questions, review the "critical thinking" questions that are presented at the end of the text chapter. Answering these questions will help you integrate important issues and themes that have been featured throughout the chapter.

1. Compare and contrast the following behaviour genetics investigations: twin studies, adoption, and family incidence studies. In what ways are these findings helpful? In what ways could these findings possibly be misinterpreted?

2. Discuss Maslow's hierarchy of needs theory. In what ways is this similar to attachment theory as proposed by Bowlby? In what ways is it different? Could these theories complement one another? Why or why not?

3. Discuss Bandura's concept of modelling. In what ways is this theory similar to Freud's concept of identification and in what way is it different? In what way do Bandura's and Freud's theories of how behaviours are learned differ from Watson's behaviourism theory?

4. Compare and contrast Freud and Erikson's theories on development. Which theory makes the most sense to you and your personal experience? Why?

5. Discuss why it is not enough to focus on one subsystem or level of analysis when viewing psychopathology. What do you gain by focusing on multifactorial causes?

ANSWER KEY

Key Terms — Matching #1

1. f	9. n	17. i
2. a	10. h	18. j
3. p	11. k	19. d
4. m	12. b	20. l
5. s	13. o	21. u
6. g	14. t	22. v
7. r	15. c	23. x
8. e	16. q	24. w

Names You Should Know

1. c	9. e
2. f	10. b
3. d	
4. a	
5. h	
6. i	
7. g	
8. j	

Key Terms — Matching #2

a. 5	g. 1	m. 3	s. 7	y. 6
b. 16	h. 20	n. 15	t. 18	
c. 25	i. 17	o. 4	u. 21	
d. 9	j. 2	p. 22	v. 19	
e. 23	k. 24	q. 13	w. 11	
f. 12	l. 10	r. 8	x. 14	

Key Terms — Matching #3

1. h	8. e	15. a	22. c
2. q	9. o	16. g	23. s
3. l	10. j	17. u	24. z
4. v	11. p	18. m	25. y
5. f	12. w	19. i	26. d
6. t	13. b	20. r	
7. n	14. k	21. x	

Key Terms — Matching #4

a. 6	f. 7	k. 8	p. 5	u. 10
b. 13	g. 2	l. 18	q. 11	v. 24
c. 1	h. 14	m. 9	r. 12	w. 15
d. 20	i. 19	n. 23	s. 16	x. 4
e. 22	j. 17	o. 21	t. 3	

Key Terms — Matching #5

1. a	4. g	7. f	10. e	13. r
2. n	5. l	8. w	11. z	14. c
3. t	6. v	9. q	12. k	15. m

16. b	19. o	22. y	24. j	26. i
17. h	20. u	23. d	25. x	
18. s	21. p			

Key Terms — Matching #6

a. 6	e. 3	i. 13	m. 20	q. 10
b. 9	f. 1	j. 19	n. 16	r. 18
c. 11	g. 17	k. 8	o. 5	s. 7
d. 15	h. 2	l. 14	p. 4	t. 12

Key Terms — Matching #7

1. h	5. r	9. p	13. k	17. g
2. l	6. m	10. a	14. q	18. j
3. e	7. t	11. c	15. o	19. s
4. n	8. b	12. d	16. f	20. i

Review of Concepts

1. false
2. discovery of the cause of general paresis; Freud; birth of psychology
3. diagnostic category
4. Penicillin
5. Biological
6. Freud
7. introspection
8. the scientific method
9. treatment
10. Humanistic
11. society
12. systems theory; biological factors; psychological factors; social factors
13. level of analysis
14. diathesis
15. cybernetics
16. receptors
17. brain
18. stroke
19. overarousal; underarousal
20. mental retardation
21. multiple genes
22. 100%; 50%
23. environmental
24. run in families
25. false
26. proximity
27. true
28. love, discipline
29. Freud; Erikson
30. problems
31. true
32. gender roles
33. dead body

Multiple Choice

1. b	6. a	11. c	16. b	21. d	26. b	31. b
2. c	7. d	12. d	17. a	22. c	27. d	32. d
3. b	8. b	13. b	18. d	23. a	28. c	
4. a	9. a	14. d	19. b	24. a	29. a	
5. c	10. b	15. c	20. a	25. b	30. a	

Understanding Research

1. marital status; ECA; thousands; mental; 1.5%; 2.4%; 4.1%; 5.8%

2. alcoholism; 8.9%; 15%; 16.2%; 24.2%; schizophrenia; every

3. causes; conflict; cause; dating; reverse causality; third variable; spurious; poverty

4. treatment policy; intervention should focus on changing the third variable; third; emotional; depression

5. factors; coefficient; –1.00 and +1.00; up; height and weight, years of education and income; down; causation

6. reverse causality, third variable; the correlation is an artifact of the relation of both variables with a third variable

7. sophistication; superior; ceremonies and cultural practices; residential schools; read and write and other practical skills; the influence of their parents; assimilate; broke up; inferior to Europeans; physical, sexual and psychological abuse.

CHAPTER 3
TREATMENT OF PSYCHOLOGICAL DISORDERS

Chapter Outline

2. Improvement Without Treatment
3. No-Treatment Control Groups
4. The Placebo Effect
    a. Placebo Control Groups
5. The Allegiance Effect
6. Efficacy and Effectiveness
7. Predictors of Psychotherapy Outcome
8. Canadian Focus: Treatments for Psychological Disorders: Research and Practice

B. Psychotherapy Process Research
1. Common Factors
2. Psychotherapy as Social Support
3. Psychotherapy as Social Influence
4. Research Close Up: Identifying Common Factors and Specific Active Ingredients

VII. Changing Social Systems: Couples, Family, and Group Therapy
A. Couples Therapy
B. Family Therapy
C. Group Therapy
D. Prevention

VIII. Specific Treatments for Specific Disorders

Learning Objectives

After reviewing the material presented in this chapter, you should be able to:

1. Understand the systems approach to psychotherapy: using different approaches for different disorders, when appropriate and effective.

2. Make broad comparisons between biological, psychodynamic, cognitive, behavioural, and humanistic approaches to treatment.

3. Distinguish the two historical trends towards spiritual/religious treatment from the natural/scientific approach to treatment.

4. Describe electroconvulsive therapy and psychosurgery as they are practiced today.

5. Evaluate the overall effectiveness of psychopharmacology in the treatment of mental illness.

6. Describe the basic goals and primary techniques involved in psychoanalysis.

7. Explain the theory behind ego analysis and the differences between psychoanalysis and psychodynamic psychotherapy.

8. Articulate the ways in which classical conditioning principles are utilized in cognitive behaviour therapy techniques as systematic desensitization, in vivo desensitization, flooding, and aversion therapy.

9. Describe contingency management and social skills training programs.

10. Understand the basic principles of attribution therapy, self-instruction training, cognitive therapy, and rational therapy.

11. Know how client-centred therapy reflects the underlying principles of humanistic psychology.

12. Describe the basic findings produced from meta-analysis of psychotherapy outcome studies.

13. Compare the efficacy research to effectiveness research on psychotherapy: what are the strengths and weaknesses of each?

14. Define psychotherapy process research and describe some of its basic findings.

15. Compare the goals, techniques, and known outcomes of couples therapy, family therapy, and group therapy; describe the differences between these approaches and individual psychotherapy.

16. List some basic recommendations that the authors suggest will improve the effectiveness of psychotherapy.

Key Terms — Matching #1

The following terms related to the treatment of psychological disorders are important to know. To test your knowledge, match the following terms with their definitions. Answers are listed at the end of the chapter.

a. Psychotherapy
b. Psychotherapy outcome research
c. Psychotherapy process research
d. Eclectic
e. Biological therapies
f. Psychodynamic therapies
g. Psychotropic drugs
h. Cognitive therapies
i. Humanistic therapies
j. Defensive style
k. Homework

l. Genuineness
m. Trephining
n. Symptom alleviation
o. Electroconvulsive therapy (ECT)
p. Bilateral ECT
q. Unilateral ECT
r. Psychosurgery
s. Prefrontal lobotomy
t. Cingulotomy
u. Psychopharmacology

1. ____ investigates similarities in practice by studying aspects of the client-therapist relationship
2. ____ an ancient form of surgery to treat mental disorders consisting of chipping a hole in the patient's skull
3. ____ treatments based on Freud's writings and later related theorists; focus on exploring the patient's past and unconscious to promote insight
4. ____ electroconvulsive therapy through both brain hemispheres
5. ____ treatments based on the perspective that mental illness is like physical illness
6. ____ a procedure in which the frontal lobes of the brain are surgically destroyed
7. ____ ability to be oneself with other people and to oneself
8. ____ treatments focusing on present feelings which encourage the client to take responsibility for their actions
9. ____ a type of therapy focused on changing the client's cognition and behaviour
10. ____ surgical destruction of specific regions of the brain
11. ____ treatment for mental illness involving the deliberate induction of a seizure by passing electricity through the brain
12. ____ electroconvulsive therapy through one brain hemisphere
13. ____ protecting oneself from being aware of inner feelings
14. ____ compares the effectiveness of alternative forms of treatment
15. ____ a form of limited psychosurgery that may be effective for very severe cases of obsessive-compulsive disorder
16. ____ the study of the use of medications to treat psychological disturbances
17. ____ the use of psychological techniques to try to produce change in the context of a special, helping relationship
18. ____ activities assigned to the client designed to continue treatment outside the therapy session
19. ____ an approach of picking different treatments according to the needs of individual disorders and individual clients
20. ____ chemical substances that affect psychological state
21. ____ reducing the dysfunctional symptoms of a disorder but not eliminating its root cause

Key Terms — Matching #2

The following terms related to the treatment of psychological disorders are important to know. To test your knowledge, match the following terms with their definitions. Answers are listed at the end of the chapter.

1. Catharsis
2. Free association
3. Psychoanalysis
4. Insight
5. Interpretation

6. Therapeutic neutrality
7. Transference
8. Countertransference
9. Psychodynamic
10. Ego analysis

11. Short-term psychodynamic psy-
    chotherapy
12. Behaviourism
13. Experiment
14. Hypothesis
15. Independent Variable
16. Experimental group
17. Control group
18. Random assignment
19. Dependent variable
20. Statistically significant
21. Confounded
22. Internal validity
23. External validity

a. _____ bringing formerly unconscious material into conscious awareness
b. _____ a form of treatment involving active focus on a particular emotional issue rather than free association, usually completed in about 25 sessions
c. _____ subjects who receive an active treatment
d. _____ an analyst's suggestion to the patient of what is the hidden meaning of his or her symptoms, dreams, or verbalizations
e. _____ the outcome that is hypothesized to vary according to the manipulations of the independent variable
f. _____ the sudden release of pent-up emotions in therapy which reduces psychic strain
g. _____ the belief that observable behaviours rather than cognitive or emotional states are the appropriate focus of psychological study
h. _____ subjects who receive no treatment or a placebo
i. _____ a purposeful stance the therapist takes of being distant and uninvolved to minimize his or her influence on free association
j. _____ changes in the dependent variable can be accurately attributed to changes in the independent variable
k. _____ a therapeutic technique where patients report without censorship whatever thoughts cross their mind, no matter how trivial
l. _____ a type of scientific investigation which can establish cause and effect
m. _____ the factor that is controlled and manipulated by the experimenter
n. _____ revisions of psychoanalysis where the therapist is more engaged anddirective and treatment is often briefer
o. _____ where the independent variable is unknowingly related to some other unmeasured factor which is not evenly distributed among the treatment groups, and this factor is causing the observed effect
p. _____ the form of psychological therapy developed by Freud
q. _____ the experimenter's specific prediction about cause and effect
r. _____ the probability that the observed difference between the groups occurred by chance alone rather than the effect of the independent variable is less than 5%
s. _____ the process whereby patients transfer their feelings about key people in their lives onto their therapist
t. _____ ensuring that each subject has a statistically equal chance of receiving different levels of the independent variable
u. _____ the process whereby therapists' feelings and reactions toward their patients affects their responses to them

v. _____ findings of an experiment can be validly generalized to other circumstances

w. _____ innovations on psychoanalytic theory giving more importance to the ego and the role of society and culture

Key Terms — Matching #3

The following terms related to the treatment of psychological disorders are important to know. To test your knowledge, match the following terms with their definitions. Answers are listed at the end of the chapter.

a. Counterconditioning
b. Systematic desensitization
c. Progressive muscle relaxation
d. Hierarchy of fears
e. In vivo desensitization
f. Flooding
g. Aversion therapy
h. Contingency management
i. Token economy
j. Social skills training
k. Assertiveness training
l. Role playing
m. Social problem solving

n. Cognitive behaviour therapy
o. Attribution retraining
p. Self-instruction training
q. Collaborative empiricism
r. Rational-emotive therapy (RET)
s. Emotional awareness
t. Client-centred therapy
u. Empathy
v. Self-disclosure
w. Unconditional positive regard
x. Gestalt therapy
y. Empty chair technique
z. Psychotherapy integration

1. _____ the therapist's description of his or her own feelings and reactions

2. _____ a technique for challenging negative distortions in thinking where the therapist gently confronts the client's fallacies and asks the client to evaluate the accuracy of his or her thinking

3. _____ teaching clients new, desirable ways of behaving that are likely to be rewarded in the everyday world

4. _____ ordering fears ranging from very mild to very frightening

5. _____ a treatment for impulsive children where an adult first models an appropriate behaviour while saying the self-instruction aloud, then the child does so, and gradually shifts from saying the self-instruction aloud to saying it silently to themselves

6. _____ nonjudgmentally valuing clients for whom they are regardless of their behaviour

7. _____ gradually being exposed to the feared stimulus in real life while simultaneously maintaining a state of relaxation

8. _____ the client has a dialogue with another part of himself or herself that is imagined sitting in an empty chair

9. _____ a humanistic therapy that follows the client's lead where the therapist offers warmth, empathy, and genuineness but the client solves his or her own problems

10. ____ an improvisational acting technique that allows clients to rehearse new social skills
11. ____ emotional understanding of others' unique feelings and perspectives
12. ____ exposure at full intensity to the feared stimulus with prevention of avoidance of the stimuli until the fear response is eliminated through extinction
13. ____ a technique of problem solving where the problem is first assessed in detail, alternative solutions are brainstormed, the different options are evaluated, one alternative is implemented, and its success is evaluated objectively
14. ____ a formalized contingency management system adopted in an institutional setting
15. ____ teaching clients to be direct about their feelings and wishes
16. ____ a cognitive behaviour therapy technique designed to directly challenge irrational beliefs about oneself and the world
17. ____ a method of inducing a calm state through the contraction and subsequent relaxation of all the major muscle groups
18. ____ trying to change how a person ascribes causes to various events in his or her life by abandoning intuitive strategies for more scientific methods
19. ____ a form of humanistic therapy that underscores affective awareness and expression, genuineness, and experiencing the moment
20. ____ a treatment for overcoming fears involving systematic exposure to imagined, feared events while simultaneously maintaining relaxation
21. ____ altering existing responses by pairing new responses with old stimuli
22. ____ pairing an unpleasant response with the stimuli that was previously sought; used for helping people stop smoking and drinking alcohol
23. ____ recognizing and experiencing true feelings
24. ____ the application of behaviour therapy into the cognitive realm
25. ____ focuses on directly changing the rewards and punishments for various behaviours: rewarding the desired behaviour and punishing the undesirable behaviour
26. ____ combining the best elements of different treatments into a unified theory of psychotherapy

Key Terms — Matching #4

The following terms related to the treatment of psychological disorders are important to know. To test your knowledge, match the following terms with their definitions. Answers are listed at the end of the chapter.

1. Outcome research
2. Process research
3. Meta-analysis
4. Spontaneous remission
5. Efficacy study
6. Effectiveness study
7. Acculturation
8. Ethnic identify
9. Conformity
10. Dissonance
11. Resistance and immersion
12. Introspection

13. Synergetic articulation and awareness
14. Placebo effect
15. Double-blind study
16. Allegiance effect
17. Couples therapy
18. Communication skills
19. Negotiation skills
20. Conflict resolution
21. Family therapy
22. Parent management training
23. Alliances
24. Group therapy
25. Psychoeducational groups
26. Experiential group therapy
27. Encounter group
28. Self-help groups
29. Community psychology
30. Primary prevention
31. Secondary prevention
32. Tertiary prevention
33. Paraprofessional

a. ____ the finding that psychotherapy researchers typically find that their favourite treatment is the most effective one

b. ____ a branch of clinical psychology that attempts to improve individual well-being by promoting social change

c. ____ correlational studies without random assignment

d. ____ teaching members of a couple effective means to resolve conflicts

e. ____ seeing intimate partners together in therapy

f. ____ experiments with randomly assigned patients in either alternative treatments or no treatment at all

g. ____ a form of experiential group therapy where members may question the self-disclosure of others when it is phoney but support honesty

h. ____ teaching members of a couple to give and take productively

i. ____ a period of conflict between self-depreciation and appreciation of one's ethnicity

j. ____ a stage of self-appreciation and ethnocentrism, accompanied by depreciation of the majority group

k. ____ designed to teach members specific information or skills relevant to psychological well-being

l. ____ studies qualities of the therapist-client relationship that predict successful outcome irrespective of the theoretical orientation of the therapist

m. ____ therapy in which the relationships among group members form the primary component of treatment

n. ____ helping members of a couple more effectively express and listen to each other's feelings and thoughts

o. ____ improving the environment in order to prevent new cases of a mental disorder from developing

p. ____ a time of self-depreciation and discrimination

q. ____ the process of learning or adopting the cultural patterns of the majority group

r. ____ neither the physician nor the patient knows whether the prescribed pill is the real medication or the placebo

s. ____ treatment of more than one unrelated person at a time

t. ____ a statistical technique that allows results from different studies to be combined in a standardized way

u. ____ a phase of questioning the basis of self-appreciation and depreciation of the majority group

v. ____ early detection of emotional problems in order to prevent them from becoming more serious and difficult to treat

w. ____ examines the result of psychotherapy; how effective it is in relieving symptoms, eliminating disorders, and improving functioning

x. ____ bringing together people who share a common problem to share information and experiences in an attempt to help themselves and on another

y. ____ therapy with two or more family members present in the session

z. ____ a type of treatment that contains no known active ingredients but is effective in some way in treating the condition

aa. ____ improvement without any treatment

bb. ____ providing intervention to an existing disorder as well as addressing some of the adverse, indirect consequences of mental illness

cc. ____ both self-appreciation and appreciation of the basis of majority group values

dd. ____ an ethnic minority member's understanding of self in terms of his or her own culture

ee. ____ strategic loyalties among family members

ff. ____ teaching parents new skills or rearing troubled children

gg. ____ people who have limited professional training but have personal experience with the problem they are treating

Names You Should Know — Matching

The following people have played an important role in the development, research, and theory of treatment for psychological disorders. To test your knowledge, match the following names with the descriptions of their contributions to the study of abnormal psychology. Answers are listed at the end of the chapter.

a. Egas Moniz
b. Joseph Breuer
c. Sigmund Freud
d. Harry Stack Sullivan
e. Erik Erikson
f. Karen Horney
g. John Bowlby

h. John B. Watson
i. Joseph Wolpe
j. Aaron Beck
k. Albert Ellis
l. Carl Rogers
m. Frederich (Fritz) Perls
n. Jerome Frank

1. ____ proposed a theory that people have conflicting ego needs to move toward, against, and away from others

2. ____ developed attachment theory

3. ____ developed client-centred therapy

4. ____ abandoned the cathartic method for free association

5. ____ an ego analyst who focused on interpersonal relationships rather than intrapsychic dynamics
6. ____ developed rational-emotive therapy
7. ____ pioneered the cathartic method
8. ____ investigated the common factors of different psychotherapies
9. ____ developed behaviourism
10. ____ won a Nobel Prize for discovering prefrontal lobotomy
11. ____ developed a cognitive behaviour therapy for depression
12. ____ developed Gestalt therapy
13. ____ developed systematic desensitization
14. ____ developed a psychosocial stage theory of development

Review of Concepts — Fill in the Blank and True/False

This section will help focus your studying by testing whether you understand the concepts presented in the text. After you have read and reviewed the material, test your comprehension and memory by filling in the following blanks or circling the right answer. Answers are listed at the end of the chapter.

1. There are hundreds of different types of psychotherapy: **true** **false**

2. The surgical removal of sexual organs was one biological treatment used for emotional problems in the past: **true** **false**

3. The development of ECT originated in attempts to treat schizophrenia that were based on the incorrect conclusion that schizophrenia was rare among people who had _____.

4. Which type of ECT produces less memory loss: **unilateral** **bilateral**

5. Which type of ECT is more effective: **unilateral** **bilateral**

6. Research has shown electroconvulsive therapy to be quite effective in treating what type of mental illness?_____

7. Psychosurgery is a reversible treatment: **true** **false**

8. What percentage of people treated with prefrontal lobotomy died?
   1-2%   **11%**   **25%**

9. What was the number one selling prescription medication for any type of ailment in the 1990's?_____

10. What was the number one selling prescription medication for any type of ailment in the 1970's? _____

11. Uncovering unconscious material and sharing the _____ view of their intrapsychic life is necessary for cure according to psychoanalysis.

12. Why is timing so important in interpreting the patient's dynamics to him or her in psychoanalysis? _____

13. Psychoanalysis is thought to be more effective for what types of disorders?

    _____

14. Sullivan hypothesized that there are two basic dimensions of interpersonal relationships: _____ and _____

15. Horney stressed the need for a person to have _____ among the three styles in which they relate to others.

16. Research shows that systematic desensitization is an effective form of treatment for fears and phobias: **true   false**

17. Research shows that aversion therapy is effective in the long-term alleviation of substance use: **true   false**

18. What is the shortcoming of the use of token economies? _____

    _____

19. Attribution retraining is effective for what type of mental disorder?

    _____

20. One of the main strengths of the behaviour therapy approach is its focus on demonstrating its effectiveness through _____

21. Humanistic psychotherapists are very active in directing therapy: **true   false**

22. When a client in Gestalt therapy is phoney, the therapist is _____

23. There is no research evidence that psychotherapy works: **true   false**

24. Research has documented that psychotherapy is more effective in treating mental disorders than chemotherapy is in treating breast cancer: **true   false**

25. What proportion of people improve without any treatment: one quarter **one third** **two thirds**

26. The quickest improvements in therapy occur in the first several months of therapy: **true** **false**

27. What does YAVIS stand for? _____

_____

28. Cognitive behaviour therapy may be more effective in the treatment of _____

29. In the classic study by Sloane and colleagues comparing behaviour therapy and psychodynamic psychotherapy, both forms of therapy were more effective than no treatment, but were not significantly different from each other: **true** **false**

30. In that same study, the single most important aspect of both types of therapy for the client was his or her _____.

31. The "file drawer problem" refers to the scientist hesitating before _____ findings that contradict their expectation.

32. Potent placebo effects have been demonstrated in cancer treatment and in surgery: **true** **false**

33. All forms of therapy emphasize the importance of _____ in the therapist-client relationship.

34. According to family systems therapists, a well-functioning family is one where the primary alliance is between _____.

35. One shortcoming of self-help groups is the lack of _____.

Multiple Choice Questions

The following multiple choice questions will test your comprehension of the material presented in the chapter. Answers are listed at the end of the chapter.

1) According to attribution theory, depressed people often attribute _____ to themselves and _____ to others.

a. success; failure
b. failure; success
c. irrational beliefs; rational beliefs
d. rational beliefs; irrational beliefs

2) Treatment outcome researchers widely accept the finding that approximately
_____ of clients improve as a result of psychotherapy.

   a. one-third   c. one-quarter
   b. two-thirds   d. one-half

3) Empathy involves:

   a. trying to put yourself in someone else's shoes in order to understand their feelings
      and perspectives
   b. trying to understand the aetiology of someone else's behaviour
   c. feeling sorry for someone because of their life situation
   d. all of the above

4) The "placebo effect" is treatment:

   a. in which the client has a dialogue with an imagined part of himself or herself
   b. in which the client is taught relaxation skills for the condition being evaluated
   c. that contains no "special ingredient" for treating the condition being evaluated
   d. which involves full intensity exposure to feared stimuli

5) Every day that Sally completes all of her chores at home her mother gives her a star.
After Sally has accumulated 15 stars, her mother will take her out for ice cream. Her
mother is most likely using which of the following to get Sally to do her chores?

   a. token economy   c. in vivo desensitization
   b. counterconditioning   d. classical conditioning

6) Which of the following would most likely ask a patient to do homework?

   a. a biological therapist   c. a humanistic therapist
   b. a psychodynamic therapist   d. a cognitive behaviour therapist

7) The following is a/are possible side effect(s) of electroconvulsive therapy (ECT):

   a. fractures   c. long-term memory loss
   b. death   d. all of the above

8) All of the following are examples of cognitive behaviour therapy EXCEPT:

   a. flooding   c. aversion therapy
   b. social skills training   d. empty chair technique

9) An experiment has internal validity if:

   a. the findings can be generalized to other circumstances
   b. changes in the dependent variable can be accurately attributed to changes in
      the independent variable

c. the researcher can control all aspects of the experimental environment

d. the researcher is able to control and manipulate the dependent variable

10) This type of therapy is primarily used to treat substance abuse disorders such as alcoholism and cigarette smoking.

    a. cognitive therapy   c. aversion therapy

    b. psychodynamic therapy   d. contingency therapy

11) Sam is a first-year college student who is extremely afraid of heights. He entered therapy after failing his first semester chemistry course because it was located on the fifth floor of a building, and Sam was too afraid to go the fifth floor to attend class. Sam's therapist gradually exposes Sam to increasing heights while having Sam simultaneously maintain a state of relaxation. Sam's therapist is using which technique to help Sam alleviate his fear of heights?

    a. in vivo desensitization   c. flooding

    b. systematic desensitization   d. counterconditioning

12) Albert Ellis is to _____ as Aaron Beck is to _____.

    a. client-centred therapy; ego analysis

    b. ego analysis; client-centred therapy

    c. rational-emotive therapy; cognitive therapy

    d. cognitive therapy; rational-emotive therapy

13) According to Sigmund Freud, all of the following are ways to reveal aspects of the unconscious mind EXCEPT:

    a. slips of the tongue   c. dreams

    b. countertransference   d. free association

14) One major difference in technique between humanistic and cognitive behaviour therapists is:

    a. humanistic psychotherapists view the nature of the therapist-client relationship differently than behaviour therapists

    b. humanistic psychotherapists focus on the patients' past and present interpersonal relationships

    c. humanistic psychotherapists focus on treatment irrespective of its causes

    d. none of the above

15) All of the following have caused a decline in the practice of classical psychoanalysis EXCEPT:

    a. the substantial amount of time required

    b. the accessibility of treatment only by those who are relatively financially secure

c. research has proven classical Freudian psychoanalysis to be ineffective

d. the limited data available on the outcome of treatment

16) In the 1990s this medication has outsold every prescription medication, including all medications used to treat physical ailments.

a. Valium

b. Prozac

c. Ritalin

d. Lithium

17) All of the following can be viewed as goals of psychoanalysis EXCEPT:

a. to rid the patient of his or her defences

b. to increase self-understanding

c. to bring unconscious material into conscious awareness

d. to release pent-up emotions and unexpressed feelings

18) Pavlov is to _____ as Skinner is to _____.

a. in vivo desensitization; systematic desensitization

b. systematic desensitization; in vivo desensitization

c. operant conditioning; classical conditioning

d. classical conditioning; operant conditioning

19) Psychotherapy outcome research indicates that:

a. clients who are young, attractive, verbal, intelligent, and successful tend to improve more in psychotherapy

b. if psychotherapy is going to be effective, it will be effective rather quickly

c. psychotherapy is generally effective when compared with no treatment at all

d. all of the above

20) Aversion therapy is a type of _____ technique.

a. classical conditioning

b. operant conditioning

c. cognitive/behaviour

d. social skills training

21) Collaborative empiricism involves:

a. relieving a client's symptoms through the use of medication

b. revealing aspects of a client's unconscious drives and conflicts

c. role-playing and assertiveness training

d. challenging a client's negative distortions

22) _____ is one of the earliest examples of a spiritual or religious tradition of healing.

a. Taboo death

b. Exorcism

c. Trephining

d. Stoning

23) Research indicates that _____ is the most effective approach to treating psychological disorders

    a. humanistic psychotherapy
    b. psychodynamic psychotherapy
    c. cognitive behaviour therapy
    d. research generally reveals few differences among approaches

24) The term "unconditional positive regard" refers to:

    a. valuing a client for who they are and refraining from judging them
    b. making positive comments to a client and never devaluing them as a person
    c. the relationship between the client and therapist
    d. none of the above

25) _____ has been the most promising avenue of biological treatment.

    a. Psychosurgery   c. Operant conditioning
    b. Classical conditioning   d. Psychopharmacology

26) In order for a finding to be statistically significant, it would need to occur by chance alone in less than:

    a. 1 out of every 5 experiments   c. 1 out of every 15 experiments
    b. 1 out of every 10 experiments d. 1 out of every 20 experiments

27) _____ is used in training clients to use relaxation techniques to cope with thoughts, feelings, or situations that provoke anxiety.

    a. Progressive relaxation   c. Applied relaxation
    b. Specific muscle relaxation d. Primary relaxation

28) This method became the cornerstone of Freud's psychoanalysis.

    a. free association   c. catharsis
    b. hypnosis   d. interpretation

29) You are more likely to receive treatment for a psychological disorder if you are diagnosed with _____ and live in _____.

    a. depression; the U.S.   c. alcohol abuse; the U.S.
    b. depression; Canada   d. alcohol abuse; Canada

Understanding Research — Fill in the Blank

Identifying Common Factors and Isolating Specific Treatments: The text presents a detailed description of a study by Borkovec and Costello in the Research Close-Up. Finding the answers to these questions will help you get a good understanding of this study and why it is important. It is not necessary to memorize the answers; the process of finding them in the textbook will help you learn the material you need to know.

1. This is an example of psychotherapy _____ research. The researchers were looking at the effectiveness of types of _____therapy in treating generalized _____ disorder. What were the two types of behaviour therapy used? _____ and _____. What was the third type used? _____ Why did they include ND? _____ _____. How many sessions were involved? _____

2. How many clients were in the study? _____ How were the clients assigned to treatment group? _____ Who supervised the ND cases? _____ How were the sessions monitored? _____ What were the four times that clients were measured? _____ _____ When were no differences among the groups found? _____ What two groups were doing much better right after treatment? _____ A year after treatment, _____% of the CBT group was functioning in the normal range of _____, while _____% of the AR and _____% of the ND clients were.

3. This study showed that both _____ and _____ were important to treatment outcome. The best predictor of successful outcome in all three groups was the client's expectation for _____.

The Experiment: The text discusses this type of research in the Research Methods section. Finding the answers to these questions will help you get a good understanding of these issues.

4. Why is the experiment the most powerful of all scientific methods? _____ What are the two types of variables? the _____ variable and the _____ variable In the example given, what are the three groups of the independent variable? Patients receiving _____ or _____. Why is random assignment to these three groups essential? _____

    _____

5. Why is the dependent variable named that? _____ _____. What is one limitation of experiments? What example of this shortcoming is given?_____ _____ What are two types of threats to internal validity? What does external validity mean?

    _____

BRIEF ESSAY

As a final exercise, write out answers to the following brief essay questions. Then compare your answers with the material presented in the text.

After you have answered these questions, review the "critical thinking" questions that are presented at the end of the text chapter. Answering these questions will help you integrate important issues and themes that have been featured throughout the chapter.

1. Compare and contrast the biological, psychodynamic, cognitive behavioural, and humanistic approaches to treating psychological disorders. In what ways might they be similar in working with a depressed patient? In what ways might they be different?

2. Discuss how the ideas of ego analysts differ from the original ideas of Freud. In what ways are they still similar?

3. What are some of the trends in psychotherapy research in Canada? Discuss some of the issues that psychotherapy researchers are currently facing in Canada.

ANSWER KEY

Key Terms — Matching #1

1. c	8. i	15. t
2. m	9. h	16. u
3. f	10. r	17. a
4. p	11. o	18. k
5. e	12. q	19. d
6. s	13. j	20. g
7. l	14. b	21. n

Names You Should Know

1. f	8. n
2. g	9. h
3. l	10. a
4. c	11. j
5. d	12. m
6. k	13. i
7. b	14. e

Matching #2

a. 4	g. 12	m. 15	s. 7
b. 11	h. 17	n. 9	t. 18
c. 16	i. 6	o. 21	u. 8
d. 5	j. 22	p. 3	v. 23
e. 19	k. 2	q. 14	w. 10
f. 1	l. 13	r. 20	

Matching #3

1. v	8. y	15. k	22. g
2. q	9. t	16. r	23. s
3. j	10. l	17. c	24. n
4. d	11. u	18. o	25. h
5. p	12. f	19. x	26. z
6. w	13. m	20. b	
7. e	14. i	21. a	

Matching #4

a. 16	h. 19	o. 30	v. 31	cc. 13
b. 29	i. 10	p. 9	w. 1	dd. 8
c. 6	j. 11	q. 7	x. 28	ee. 23
d. 20	k. 25	r. 15	y. 21	ff. 22
e. 17	l. 2	s. 24	z. 14	gg. 33
f. 5	m. 26	t. 3	aa. 4	
g. 27	n. 18	u. 12	bb. 32	

Multiple Choice

1. b	3. a	5. a	7. d	9. b	11. a	13. b	15. c
2. b	4. c	6. d	8. d	10. c	12. c	14. a	16. b

17. a   19. d   21. d   23. d   25. d   27. c   29. b
18. d   20. a   22. c   24. a   26. d   28. a

Review of Concepts

1. true
2. true
3. epilepsy
4. unilateral
5. bilateral
6. severe depression
7. false
8. 25%
9. Prozac
10. Valium
11. analyst's
12. premature interpretations will be rejected—too threatening
13. milder forms of depression and anxiety
14. power and closeness
15. balance
16. true
17. false
18. they do not generalize to uncontrolled environments
19. depression
20. research
21. false
22. confrontational
23. false
24. true
25. one third
26. true
27. young, attractive, verbal, intelligent, and successful
28. anxiety
29. true
30. relationship with the therapist
31. publishing
32. true
33. warmth
34. the parents
35. research on process and outcome

Understanding Research

1. outcome; behaviour; anxiety; Applied relaxation and Cognitive behaviour therapy; Nondirective therapy; to control for common factors; 12

2. 55; randomly; an expert nondirective therapist; audiotape; immediately before and after therapy, 6 months and 1 year after therapy; before therapy; AR and CBT; 58%; anxiety; 37%; 28%

3. specific treatment factors; common factors; success

4. It can determine cause and effect; independent; dependent; medication; psychotherapy; no treatment; to ensure that differences among groups are caused by the independent variable and not selection bias

5. It is hypothesized to depend on the independent variable; interesting variables cannot always be manipulated practically or ethically; whether abusive parenting causes psychological problems; the independent variable could be manipulated poorly or it could be confounded with other variables; whether the findings can be generalized to the real world.

CHAPTER 4
CLASSIFICATION AND ASSESSMENT OF ABNORMAL BEHAVIOUR

Chapter Outline

I.   Overview

II. Basic Issues in Classification
      A. Categories versus Dimensions
      B. From Description to Theory

III. Classification of Abnormal Behaviour
      A. Brief Historical Perspective
      B. The DSM-IV System
          1. Diagnostic Axes
          2. Other Domains for Assessment
      C. Culture-Bound Syndromes

IV. Evaluation of Classification Systems
      A. Reliability
      B. Validity
      C. Unresolved Questions
      D. Problems and Limitations of the DSM-IV System
      E. Research Methods: Diagnostic Reliability

V.   Basic Issues in Assessment
      A. The Purposes of Clinical Assessment
      B. Assumptions about Behaviour
          1. Consistency of Behaviour
          2. Levels of Analysis
      C. Evaluating the Utility of Assessment Procedures

VI. Assessment Procedures
      A. Assessment of Psychological Systems
          1. Interviews
              a. Structured Interviews
              b. Advantages
              c. Limitations
          2. Observational Procedures
              a. Rating Scales
              b. Behavioural Coding Systems
              c. Advantages
              d. Limitations

3. Personality Tests and Self-Report Inventories
    a. Personality Inventories
    b. Advantages
    c. Limitations
    d. Other Self-Report Inventories
4. Projective Personality Tests
    a. Advantages
    b. Limitations
B. Assessment of Social Systems
C. Assessment of Biological Systems
    1. Psychophysiological Assessment
        a. Advantages
        b. Limitations
    2. Brain Imaging Techniques
        a. Static Brain Imaging
        b. Dynamic Brain Imaging
        c. Advantages
        d. Limitations

Learning Objectives

After reviewing the material presented in this chapter, you should be able to:

1. Define classification system, assessment, and diagnosis.

2. Distinguish between a categorical approach to classification and a dimensional approach.

3. Explain why DSM-III represented a turning point in the diagnosis of psychiatric disorders.

4. Describe the five axes used in diagnosis in DSM-IV.

5. Know the meaning and implications of reliability and validity in diagnosis and classification.

6. Give some of the advantages and also limitations of interview data for purposes of assessment.

7. Compare the three types of observational procedures—informal observations, rating scales, and behavioural coding systems.

8. Describe the strengths and weaknesses of the MMPI-2.

9. List some of the advantages as well as limitations of using projective tests for assessment and diagnosis.

10. Know the two methods employed for the assessment of social systems.

11. Describe two uses of psychophysiological assessment procedures and two limitations of this approach.

12. Compare static brain imaging techniques with dynamic brain imaging techniques in terms of the type of data each provides.

Key Terms — Matching #1

The following terms related to classification and assessment are important to know. To test your knowledge, match the following terms with their definitions. Answers are listed at the end of the chapter.

a. Assessment
b. Diagnosis
c. Classification system
d. Categorical approach
e. Dimensional approach
f. Stigma
g. Phenylketonuria (PKU)
h. Dementia praecox
i. Manic-depressive psychosis
j. Diagnostic and Statistical Manual of Mental Disorders (DSM)
k. International Classification of Diseases (ICD)
l. Labelling theory

m. Multiaxial classification
n. Inclusion criteria
o. Exclusion criteria
p. Reliability
q. Inter-rater reliability
r. Validity
s. Kappa
t. Etiological validity
u. Concurrent validity
v. Predictive validity
w. Comorbidity
x. Test-retest reliability
y. Split-half reliability

1. ____ an old term for what we now call schizophrenia
2. ____ a system for grouping together objects or organisms that share certain properties
3. ____ a system in which the person is rated with regard to several separate aspects of behaviour or adjustment
4. ____ the process of gathering and organizing information about a person's behaviour
5. ____ looks at the social context in which abnormal behaviour occurs; sees mental disorders as maladaptive social roles
6. ____ assumes that distinctions between members of different categories are qualitative
7. ____ concerned with factors that contribute to the onset of the disorder
8. ____ the diagnostic system for mental disorders published by the World Health Organization
9. ____ describes the objects of classification in terms of continuous dimensions

10. ____ concerned with the present time and with correlations between the disorder and other symptoms, circumstances, and test procedures
11. ____ the simultaneous appearance of two or more disorders in the same person
12. ____ an old term for what we now call bipolar mood disorder
13. ____ the diagnostic system for mental disorders published by the American Psychiatric Association
14. ____ symptoms or characteristic features that must be present in order for a person to meet the diagnostic criteria for a particular disorder
15. ____ the identification or recognition of a disorder on the basis of its characteristic symptoms
16. ____ an inherited metabolic disorder that, uncontrolled, produces mental retardation
17. ____ symptoms or conditions that are used to rule out the presence of a particular disorder
18. ____ a statistic of reliability that reflects the proportion of agreement that occurred above and beyond what would have occurred by chance alone
19. ____ the meaning or systematic importance of a construct or measurement
20. ____ the consistency of measurements over time
21. ____ a label that sets the person apart from others in a negative way
22. ____ concerned with the future and with the stability of the problem over time
23. ____ agreement among clinicians
24. ____ the internal consistency of items within a test
25. ____ the consistency of measurements

Key Terms — Matching #2

The following terms related to classification and assessment are important to know. To test your knowledge, match the following terms with their definitions. Answers are listed at the end of the chapter.

1 Structured interviews
2. Informal observations
3. Rating Scales
4. Behavioural coding systems
5. Self-monitoring
6. Reactivity
7. Personality tests
8. Personality inventories
9. Minnesota Multiphasic Personality Inventory
10. Validity scales
11. Actuarial interpretation
12. Beck Depression Inventory
13. Self-report inventories
14. Projective tests
15. Rorschach test
16. Thematic Apperception Test
17. Camberwell Family Interview
18. Family Environment Scale
19. Family Interaction Coding System
20. Computerized topographic scanning
21. Magnetic resonance imaging
22. Positron emission tomography
23. Single photon emission computed tomography
24. Basal ganglia
25. Yale-Brown Obsessive Compulsive Scale

a. ____ a procedure where clients record their own behaviour
b. ____ analysis of test results based on an explicit set of rules derived from empirical research
c. ____ objective tests consisting of a series of straightforward statements that the person indicates how true or false they are in relation to himself or herself
d. ____ a projective test also known as the inkblot test
e. ____ a static brain imaging technique which passes X-rays through brain tissue to measure the density of the tissue
f. ____ a dynamic brain imaging technique using special radioactive elements to produce relatively detailed images of the brain, which can reflect changes in brain activity as a person performs various tasks
g. ____ personality tests in which the person is asked to interpret a series of ambiguous stimuli
h. ____ focus on the frequency of specific behavioural events, requiring fewer inferences on the part of the observer
i. ____ a self-report inventory designed to measure social characteristics of families
j. ____ a brain imaging technique which passes electromagnetic phenomena through brain tissue to provide a static image of brain structures
k. ____ an objective personality inventory aimed at a focal topic or at one aspect of a person's adjustment
l. ____ people altering their behaviour, either intentionally or unintentionally, when they know they are being observed
m. ____ a self-report inventory used as an index of severity of depression
n. ____ standardized situations where a person's behaviour can be sampled, and reflects on underlying abilities or personality traits
o. ____ a coding system for observations of interactions between parents and children in their homes
p. ____ an assessment interview that follows a specific question-and-answer format
q. ____ a projective test consisting of a series of drawings that depict human figures in various ambiguous situations
r. ____ reflect the person's attitude toward the test and the openness and consistency with which the questions were answered
s. ____ an assessment device where the observer makes judgments that place the person along a dimension
t. ____ a dynamic brain imaging technique using single-photon-emitting compounds
u. ____ a structured interview designed to measure expressed emotion in families
v. ____ a part of the thalamus implicated in obsessions and compulsions
w. ____ a very widely used personality inventory with a true-false format that produces scores on ten clinical scales and four validity scales
x. ____ qualitative observations of a person's behaviour and/or environment with no attempt to quantify the observed characteristics
y. ____ an interview-based rating scale used extensively to assess obsessions and compulsions

Names You Should Know — Matching

The following people have played an important role in the classification and assessment of mental disorders. To test your knowledge, match the following names with the descriptions of their contributions to the study of abnormal psychology. Answers are listed at the end of the chapter.

a. Emil Kraepelin   b. Thomas Scheff   c. Hermann Rorschach

1. _____ a proponent of labelling theory
2. _____ pioneered the type of categorical classification system currently used
3. _____ developed the best-known projective test, the inkblot test

Review of Concepts — Fill in the Blank and True/False

This section will help focus your studying by testing whether you understand the concepts presented in the text. After you have read and reviewed the material, test your comprehension and memory by filling in the following blanks or circling the right answer. Answers are listed at the end of the chapter.

1. In the field of psychopathology, assigning a diagnosis implies the etiology of the person's problem: **true**   **false**

2. Classification systems can be based on descriptive or _____ similarities.

3. Which type of emphasis typically comes first in the development of scientific classification systems?   **aetiological factors**   **description**

4. What were three criticisms of psychiatric classification systems during the 1950s and 1960s? _____,

_____,

and _____.

5. The major change that occurred in the third edition of the DSM was a focus on clinical description rather than on _____.

6. Labelling theory views symptoms of mental disorders as violations of residual _____.

7. Labelling theory predicts that people from lower status groups, like the impoverished are   **more**   or   **less**   likely to receive a diagnosis.

8. The authors of your text conclude that labelling theory provides a good account for abnormal behaviour: **true   false**

9. How many diagnostic axes are there in the DSM-IV? _____

10. The presence of general medical conditions are coded on one of the axes of a DSM-IV diagnosis: **true   false**

11. One example of a culture-bound syndrome, amok, is found among mostly men in Malaysia and consists of a period of brooding and paranoid thinking followed by an angry, aggressive outburst in response to a perceived _____.

12. Clinicians have been more willing to drop old categories in revisions of the DSM than to include new categories: **true   false**

13. Comorbidity rates among mental disorders as defined in the DSM system are very low: **true   false**

14. What are the three primary goals which guide most assessment procedures?

    _____

    _____

    _____

15. The meaning or importance of an assessment procedure is known as its:
    reliability   validity

16. There are only a few select assessment procedures available to clinicians today:
    true   false

17. Clinical interviews provide clinicians with the opportunity to assess a person's appearance and nonverbal behaviour: **true   false**

18. Clinical interviews are either structured or_____.

19. One advantage of structured interviews is that anybody can conduct them, saving the expense of a clinician's time: **true   false**

20. Clinical interviews are of limited use with young children: **true   false**

21. Observations provide a more realistic view of behaviour than do people's recollections of their actions and feelings: **true   false**

22. One problem with observational procedures is that they can be time-consuming and expensive: **true   false**

23. Why do some clinicians prefer to use the original version of the MMPI?

    _____

24. One advantage of the MMPI is that it allows the clinician to use his or her intuition in coming up with scores on the clinical scales: **true   false**

25. One unique feature of the MMPI is the   **clinical**   or   **validity**   scales.

26. Which is a more complex assessment tool?   **the MMPI   the BDI**

27. If a person scores as being significantly depressed on the Beck Depression Inventory, he or she definitely will meet diagnostic criteria for depression:
    true   false

28. The Exner system, a new scoring system for the Rorschach test, is based more on which of the following?   **content   form**

29. One strength of the original Rorschach scoring system was its high reliability:
    true   false

30. Projective tests are more likely to be used by a therapist with which type of theoretical orientation?   **psychodynamic   behavioural**

31. List three types of physiological measures that provide information about a person's psychological state: _____

    _____

32. Men who exhibit physiological responses that indicate intense arousal during discussions with their wives about marital conflicts but who do not express their arousal _____ are more likely to divorce.

33. Brain imaging techniques are used to rule out _____ as a cause of behavioural or cognitive deficits.

Multiple Choice Questions

The following multiple choice questions will test your comprehension of the material presented in the chapter. Answers are listed at the end of the chapter.

1) A definitive characteristic of ALL projective tests is:

   a. a true-false response format
   b. the use of a list of open-ended sentences that the individual must answer
   c. the use of items describing various thoughts, feelings, and behaviours that the individual must rate
   d. the use of ambiguous stimuli

2) Which approach to classification is based on an ordered sequence or on quantitative measurements rather than qualitative judgments?

   a. dimensional approach
   b. categorical approach
   c. diagnostic approach
   d. interview approach

3) Which of the following is NOT an axis of DSM-IV?

   a global rating of adaptive functioning
   b. psychosocial and environmental problems
   c. general medical conditions that may be relevant to the patient's current behaviours or that may affect treatment
   d. familial communication style

4) Which would NOT be considered a limitation of a clinical interview?

   a. the information gathered is subjective and may be influenced or distorted by errors in memory or perception
   b. the person may be reluctant to directly share with the interviewer experiences that are embarrassing or socially undesirable
   c. Interviews are expensive and time-consuming
   d. people may not be able to give a rational account of their problems due to the presence of limited verbal skills, a psychotic process, etc.

5) Analyzing a test on the basis of an explicit set of rules based on empirical research is referred to as what type of procedure?

   a. actuarial
   b. self report
   c. diagnostic
   d. cookbook

6) A criticism of psychiatric diagnosis in the 1950's and 1960's was that:

   a. the system in use was too detailed and included too many categories
   b. the system was too descriptive and did not make assumptions about aetiology

c. once labelled with a diagnosis, individuals did not receive the appropriate treatment

d. once labelled with a diagnosis, an individual might be motivated to continue to act in a manner expected from someone who is mentally ill

7) Research of psychiatric diagnosis in the 1950's and 1960's was that:

a. wives who do not express their negative emotions often display sleep difficulties

b. husbands who do not express their negative emotions often display changes in heart rate and skin conductance that indicate intense arousal

c. wives who verbally report negative emotion do not display any physiological changes

d. husbands who verbally express their negative emotions also show changes in their sleep patterns

8) Which of the following does NOT reflect a rationale for classifying abnormal behaviour?

a. a diagnostic system can be used to help clinicians more effectively communicate with one another

b. a diagnostic system can be used to organize information that may be helpful for research purposes

c. a diagnostic system can be used to label people who are socially deviant

d. a diagnostic system can be used in making management and treatment decisions

9) When an observer is asked to make judgments about some aspect of an individual's behaviour along a dimension, the observer would be using:

a. a projective instrument   c. a self-report inventory

b. a rating scale   d. a structured interview

10) Interpretation of a person's responses to the MMPI is based upon:

a. reviewing the clinical scale for which the person received the highest score

b. reading through all of the inventory items and noting how the person answered each one

c. reviewing the clinical scale for which the person received the lowest score

d. examining the pattern of scale scores, paying particular attention to those scales that have elevated scores

11) An example of a type of observational procedure would be:

a. the Rorschach test   c. a behavioural coding system

b. the MMPI   d. dynamic brain imaging

12) Which would NOT be considered a primary goal of assessment?

a. making predictions

b. reconstructing people's developmental history

c. planning interventions
d. evaluating interventions

13) An advantage of the MMPI is that:

   a. it provides information about the individual's test-taking attitude
   b. it assesses a wide range of problem areas that would take a clinician several hours to review in an interview
   c. it is scored objectively and is not influenced by the clinician's personal opinion about the individual taking the test
   d. all of the above

14) How many axes are included in the DSM-IV?

   a. 3   c. 5
   b. 4   d. 6

15) What would be considered an advantage of a structured clinical interview compared to a regular clinical interview?

   a. it provides the interviewer with a series of systematic questions that allow for the collection of important diagnostic information
   b it allows for the establishment of a better therapeutic rapport with the client
   c. it allows the interviewer flexibility in gathering information
   d. all of the above

16) Projective techniques place considerable emphasis upon which of the following?

   a. the importance of unconscious motivations such as conflicts and impulses
   b. the importance of familial values that may influence the person's behaviour
   c. the presence of symptoms, which suggest that the person has lost contact with reality and is presently psychotic
   d. the importance of the person's cultural background in understanding his or her personality

17) An example of a measure that assesses a social system is:

   a. Positron emission tomography
   b. the Family Interaction Coding System
   c. the Beck Depression Inventory
   d. the Yale-Brown Obsessive-Compulsive Scale

18) Which type of study could be used to validate a clinical syndrome?

   a. a follow-up study that demonstrated a distinctive course or outcome
   b. a family study supporting that the syndrome "breeds true"
   c. a study demonstrating an association between the clinical syndrome and an underlying biochemical abnormality
   d. all of the above

19) An advantage of psychophysiological assessment is that:

    a. these types of procedures do not depend on self-report and may be less likely to be under the person's control
    b. physiological assessment is less expensive and less time consuming than the use of personality inventories
    d. physiological procedures are frequently used in clinical settings

20) The most commonly used procedure in psychological assessment is:

    a. self-report inventories
    b. projective testing
    c. clinical interview
    d. behavioural observation

21) A limitation of brain-imaging procedures is that:

    a. brain-imaging procedures can only be used with certain populations
    b. although useful for research, brain-imaging procedures cannot be used for diagnostic purposes because norms have not yet been established
    c. brain-imaging procedures tend to give imprecise information
    d. the results of brain-imaging procedures tend to be overly responsive to outside factors such as whether the person is presently medicated

22) Which of the following problems could NOT be assessed through the use of an observational measure?

    a. hand-washing
    b. crying
    c. low self-esteem
    d. hitting, punching, or spitting at school

23) A limitation of the use of projective tests is:

    a. information obtained from projective tests tends to duplicate what can already be obtained from a clinical interview
    b. projective tests cannot be used with children
    c. projective tests cannot be used with psychotic individuals
    d. the reliability of scoring and interpretation appears to be low

24) Which type of study can be used to demonstrate the reliability of a set of diagnostic criteria?

    a. a study demonstrating that clinicians using the same set of criteria arrived at the same diagnosis for the same set of individuals
    b. a study supporting that individuals with the same diagnosis responded to the same kind of treatment
    c. a study supporting that the set of diagnostic criteria could be meaningful to other cultures when properly translated
    d. all of the above

25) The L (Lie) Scale of the MMPI is an example of which type of scale?

  a. reactivity   c. projective
  b clinical   d. validity

26) The first two axes of the DSM-IV primarily focus on which of the following?

  a. symptomatic behaviours   c. medical history
  b. amilial functioning   d. intrapsychic functioning

27) Which would NOT be considered a drawback of using a physiological assessment measure?

  a. the equipment used may be intimidating to certain people
  b. physiological responses can be influenced by many outside factors such as age and medication
  c. physiological response measures have not demonstrated adequate validity
  d. the stability of physiological response systems vary from person to person

Understanding Research — Fill in the Blank

Pibloktoq: A culture-bound syndrome: The text presents a detailed description of a culture-bound syndrome called Pibloktoq. Although finding the answers to these questions will help you get a good understanding of this study and why it is important, it is not necessary to memorize the answers; the process of finding them in the textbook will help you learn the material you need to know.

1.   The glossary of culture-bound syndromes lists unique ways a certain culture

expresses negative _____, also known as "_____."

Pibloktoq, one example of a culture-bound syndrome, is unique to

_____. Research on this syndrome has been primarily conducted by

medical anthropologists who use a combination of _____ and

_____ research methods.

2.   This syndrome involves _____ or "attacks" accompanied by

_____ and extreme _____. They usually last

between _____ minutes. The "attacks" are characterized by one or

more of the following: tearing off clothing; rapid, incoherent speech; _____;

throwing oneself in the water or snow; or throwing objects about. The sufferer and

other people are _____ harmed during one of these attacks.

Many "attacks" are preceded by a period of _____, social withdrawal, irritable mood, or stress. Several theories exist to explain pibloktoq. One proposes that the "attacks" are a socially sanctioned way of expressing _____. Another theory proposes that _____ factors may cause Pibloktoq.

3. Pibloktoq resembles the DSM _____ disorders which are characterized by a disruption in the usually integrated functions of consciousness, memory, identity, and _____. As such, Pibloktoq would be classified in DSM-IV-TR terms as a _____.

Diagnostic Reliability: The text discusses this type of research in the Research Methods section. Finding the answers to these questions will help you get a good understanding of these issues.

4. Kappa is a measure of how well clinicians agree on a diagnosis above and beyond agreement that would be expected by _____. A _____ kappa value indicates agreement is less than what would be expected by chance. What value indicates perfect agreement? _____ What is the convention for the value of kappa that is relatively good? _____ What level suggests poor agreement? _____ What category of disorder needs a lot of work to improve kappa?

    _____

5. Clinicians agree much better on the major heading of disorder than they do on the specific _____. This is like having disagreement about whether a passing vehicle is a Chrysler, Ford, or Toyota _____. The clinicians who were diagnosing in this study were _____ mental health professionals in their countries. This means that the kappa values found in this study are _____.

Brief Essay

As a final exercise, write out answers to the following brief essay questions. Then compare your answers with the material presented in the text.

After you have answered these questions, review the "critical thinking" questions that are presented at the end of the text chapter. Answering these questions will help you integrate important issues and themes that have been featured throughout the chapter.

1. Briefly discuss the major assumptions of labelling theory. Then discuss your personal position about the theory; that is, to what extent do you agree with its major points?

2. Review examples of both scientific and nonscientific factors that affect the development of diagnostic systems. When do you see nonscientific factors playing an important role in this process?

3. Describe the major purposes of clinical assessment. What are the major assumptions regarding the nature of human behaviour upon which the assessment process is based?

4. Pretend that you are a clinician who has just received a call from a potential client. The problem for which the client is seeking treatment is depression. What assessment procedures reviewed in your chapter could you use to determine whether or not the client is really depressed? What type of information would you expect to obtain from each method?

ANSWER KEY

Key Terms — Matching #1

1. h	10. u	19. r
2. c	11. w	20. x
3. m	12. i	21. f
4. a	13. j	22. v
5. l	14. n	23. q
6. d	15. b	24. y
7. t	16. g	25. p
8. k	17. o	
9. e	18. s	

Names You Should Know

1. b
2. a
3. c

Matching #2

a. 5	h. 4	o. 19	v. 24
b. 11	i. 18	p. 1	w. 9
c. 8	j. 21	q. 16	x. 2
d. 15	k. 13	r. 10	y. 25
e. 20	l. 6	s. 3	
f. 22	m. 12	t. 23	
g. 14	n. 7	u. 17	

Multiple Choice

1. d	6. d	11. c	16. a	21. b	26. a
2. a	7. b	12. b	17. b	22. c	27. c
3. d	8. c	13. d	18. d	23. d	
4. c	9. b	14. c	19. a	24. a	
5. a	10. d	15. a	20. c	25. d	

Review of Concepts

1. false
2. structural
3. description
4. lack of consistency in diagnoses among clinicians; diagnoses are problems in living, not medical disorders; labels might increase maladaptive behaviour
5. theories of psychopathology
6. rules
7. more
8. false
9. 5
10. true
11. insult
12. false
13. false
14. making predictions, planning interventions, and evaluating interventions
15. validity
16. false
17. true
18. nondirective
19. false
20. true
21. true
22. true
23. because of all the research done with it
24. false
25. validity
26. MMPI
27. false
28. form
29. false
30. psychodynamic
31. heart rate, respiration rate, and skin conductance
32. verbally
33. brain tumors

Understanding Research

1. emotion; "idioms of distress"; people living in the arctic; anthropological; clinical research

2. dissociative episodes; confusion; excitement; 5 – 60; fleeing; rarely; depression; distress or a desire to be cared for; dietary

3. dissociative; perception; dissociative disorder not otherwise specified

4. chance; negative; +1.0; .70 or above; below .40; personality disorders

5. subtype; minivan; leading; probably higher than what occurs in typical practice

CHAPTER 5
MOOD DISORDERS AND SUICIDE

Chapter Outline

I. Overview

II. Typical Symptoms and Associated Features
    A. Emotional Symptoms
    B. Cognitive Symptoms
    C. Somatic Symptoms
    D. Behavioural Symptoms
    E. Other Problems Commonly Associated with Depression

III. Classification
    A. Brief Historical Perspective
    B. Contemporary Diagnostic Systems
       1. Unipolar Disorders
       2. Bipolar Disorders
       3. Further Descriptions and Subtypes
    C. Course and Outcome
       1. Unipolar Disorders
       2. Bipolar Disorders

IV. Epidemiology
    A. Incidence and Prevalence
    B. Gender Differences
    C. Cross-Cultural Differences
    D. Risk for Mood Disorders Across the Life Span
    E. Comparisons Across Generations

V. Etiological Considerations and Research
    A. Social Factors
       1. Stressful Life Events and Unipolar Disorders
       2. Social Factors and Bipolar Disorders
    B. Psychological Factors
       1. Cognitive Responses to Failure and Disappointment
          a. Theoretical Proposals
          b. Research Evidence
       2. Interpersonal Factors and Social Skills
          a. Social Relationships
          b. Response Styles and Gender
       3. Integration of Cognitive and Interpersonal Factors

C. Biological Factors
   1. Genetics
      a. Family Studies
      b. Twin Studies
      c. Genetic Risk and Sensitivity to Stress
      d. Mode of Transmission and Linkage Studies
   2. Neurotransmitters and Depression
   3. The Neuroendocrine System
   4. Brain Imaging Studies
D. The Interaction of Social, Psychological, and Biological Factors

VI. Treatment
   A. Unipolar Disorders
      1. Cognitive Therapy
      2. Interpersonal Therapy
      3. Antidepressant Medications
         a. Selective Serotonin Reuptake Inhibitors
         b. Tricyclics
         c. Monoamine Oxidase Inhibitors
      4. The Efficacy of Psychotherapy and Medication
   B. Bipolar Disorders
      a. Lithium
      b. Anticonvulsant Medications
      c. Psychotherapy
   C. Electroconvulsive Therapy
   D. Seasonal Mood Disorders

VII. Suicide
   A. Classification of Suicide
   B. Epidemiology of Suicide
   C. Aetiology of Suicide
      1. Psychological Factors
      2. Biological Factors
      3. Social Factors
   D. Treatment of Suicidal People
      1. Crisis Centres and Hot Lines
      2. Psychotherapy with Suicidal Clients
      3. Medication
      4. Involuntary Hospitalization

Learning Objectives

After reviewing the material presented in this chapter, you should be able to:

1. Distinguish clinical depression from a depressed mood.

2. Define emotion, affect, mood, depression, and mania.

3. Identify the major emotional, cognitive, and somatic symptms involved in depression.

4. Contrast major depressive disorder with dysthymia.

5. Distinguish bipolar I, bipolar II, and cyclothymia.

6. Know the average age of onset for depression and bipolar disorder, as well as the typical recovery rates for each disorder.

7. Understand how social factors, especially interpersonal loss, can be influential in the development of depression.

8. Contrast Beck's cognitive model with the hopelessness model of depression.

9. Appreciate the interaction between social, psychological, and biological factors in the development and maintenance factors in the development and maintenance of mood disorders.

10. Compare interpersonal therapy with cognitive therapy approaches.

11. Compare the effectiveness of cognitive therapy, interpersonal therapy, and antidepressant medication with a placebo control group in the treatment of depression.

12. Understand the pros and cons of electroconvulsive shock therapy.

13. Comprehend Durkheim's basic theory about suicide and identify the four types of suicide he delineated.

14. Have a basic understanding of the aetiology, epidemiology, and treatment of suicidal ideation and suicidal behaviour.

Key Terms — Matching

The following terms related to mood disorders are important to know. To test your knowledge, match the following terms with their definitions. Answers are listed at the end of the chapter.

a.   Emotion
b.   Affect
c.   Mood
d.   Depression
e.   Depressed mood

f.   Clinical depression
g.   Mania
h.   Mood disorders
i.   Unipolar mood disorder
j.   Bipolar mood disorder

k.	Manic-depressive disorder	q.	Dysthymia
l.	Dysphoria	r.	Hypomania
m.	Euphoria	s.	Cyclothymia
n.	Somatic symptoms	t.	Melancholia
o.	Psychomotor retardation	u.	Seasonal affective disorder
p.	Comorbidity	v.	Double depression

1. ____ a mood disorder with onset of episodes associated with changes in the seasons
2. ____ a state of incredible well-being and elation
3. ____ a term for a mood or a clinical syndrome that involves sadness, despair, and disappointment
4. ____ a combination of major depression and dysthymia
5. ____ chronic, mild depression lasting for at least two years
6. ____ observable behaviours associated with a person's feelings
7. ____ having more than one mental disorder at the same time
8. ____ a disturbance in mood which can include elation, decreased need for sleep, pressured speech, inflated self-esteem
9. ____ symptoms related to bodily functions, like sleep and appetite disturbance
10. ____ an especially severe form of depression
11. ____ subjective states of feeling, often accompanied by physiological changes
12. ____ a category of mental disorders involving episodes of disturbance of mood, characterized either by clinical depression or mania
13. ____ chronic, mild form of bipolar disorder with episodes of hypomania and depression lasting at least two years
14. ____ a pervasive, long-standing emotional response that affects a person's perception of their world
15. ____ a classification of mood disorder involving periods of depression only
16. ____ a classification of mood disorder involving periods of depression and mania, or sometimes mania alone
17. ____ a mood state involving sadness and despair that is not a psychiatric syndrome
18. ____ the former term for bipolar disorder
19. ____ a psychiatric syndrome involving sadness and despair as well as fatigue, sleep disturbance, loss of energy, or changes in appetite
20. ____ a state of depression, despondency, sadness
21. ____ an episode of increased energy that is not as extreme as mania
22. ____ significant slowing of movements or speech

Key Terms — Matching #2

The following terms related to mood disorders are important to know. To test your knowledge, match the following terms with their definitions. Answers are listed at the end of the chapter.

1. Remission
2. Relapse
3. Neurasthenia
4. Schema
5. Learned helplessness theory
6. Hopelessness
7. Catecholamine hypothesis
8. Indolamine hypothesis
9. Hypothalamic-pituitary-adrenal axis
10. Dexamethasone suppression test
11. Analogue studies
12. Tricyclics
13. Monoamine oxidase inhibitors
14. Selective serotonin reuptake inhibitors
15. Lithium carbonate
16. Electroconvulsive therapy

a. _____ studies that focus on behaviours that are similar to mental disorders, or features of mental disorders; often animal models of psychopathology

b. _____ a theory that depression is associated with lowered levels and mania with an excess of catecholamines, particularly norepinephrine, in the brain

c. _____ a category of antidepressant medication which must not be taken with certain foods, especially cheese and chocolate

d. _____ a theory that depression may be related to a person's expectation that good things will not happen and bad things will, regardless of his or her actions

e. _____ a lasting and highly organized cognitive structure that influences how people perceive and interpret events in their environment

f. _____ a period of recovery from a mental disorder

g. _____ a diagnostic term referring to multiple complaints involving physical symptoms, such as headaches and weakness

h. _____ a medication often used to treat bipolar disorder

i. _____ a theory that depression is associated with abnormalities in levels of serotonin in the central nervous system

j. _____ a pathway in the endocrine system that regulates hormone secretions by the adrenal glands; may be involved in the aetiology of depression

k. _____ a series of treatments in which electric current is run through the patient's brain; effective in the treatment of severe depression

l. _____ the return of active symptoms in a person who had recovered from a previous episode

m. _____ used to study endocrine dysfunction in people with mood disorders; half of depressed patients show an abnormal response to this test

n. _____ a new class of antidepressants which have fewer side effects than older medications

o. _____ an older class of antidepressants which benefit many depressed people

p. _____ a theory that depression is like the passive behaviour of animals exposed to uncontrollable electric shock, that depressed people do not see a relations between their behaviour and events that occur in their lives

Names You Should Know — Matching

The following people have played an important role in research and theory of mood disorders. To test your knowledge, match the following names with the descriptions of their contributions to the study of abnormal psychology. Answers are listed at the end of the chapter.

a. Aaron Beck
b. James Coyne
c. Emile Durkheim

d. Emil Kraeplin
e. Peter Lewinsohn
f. Martin Seligman

1. ____ conceptualized depression as cognitive in origin, arising from distortions, errors, and biases common in the thinking of depressed people
2. ____ identified four types of suicide based on the type of society in which the person lives
3. ____ proposed the first classification system for mental disorders, dividing them into dementia praecox and manic-depressive psychosis
4. ____ proposed the interpersonal perspective of depression, where depressed people's behaviour drives away important people in their lives
5. ____ proposed a behavioural model of depression where adaptive behaviour is not positively reinforced by the environment and therefore decreases
6. ____ proposed the learned helplessness model of depression

Review of Concepts — Fill in the Blank and True/False

This section will help focus your studying by testing whether you understand the concepts presented in the text. After you have read and reviewed the material, test your comprehension and memory by filling in the following blanks or circling the right answer. Answers are listed at the end of the chapter.

1. Major depression is the leading cause of disability worldwide: **true   false**

2. Many depressed and manic patients are irritable: **true   false**

3. People who are depressed often have trouble with their thinking: they have trouble _____, and can't make _____.

4. The depressive triad is typical of depressed patients: they focus on the negative aspects of 1) _____, 2) _____, and 3) _____.

5. People with _____ can be easily distracted, incoherent, and grandiose.

6. People with _____ can be preoccupied with thoughts of suicide and may actually make a suicide attempt that may be successful.

7. Sometimes depressed people have trouble falling asleep and wake up throughout the night or very early in the morning, but it is much more common for a depressed person to sleep much more than usual: **true**   **false**

8. Depressed people typically eat more than usual: **true**   **false**

9. People with _____ are less likely to initiate sexual activity and people with _____ are more likely to do so.

10. List three types of disorders that have high comorbidity with mood disorders (and are also found in higher rates than expected among relatives of people with mood disorders): _____, _____, and _____.

11. Some people with mood disorders become psychotic (lose touch with reality, experience hallucinations and delusions) during their episodes of depression or mania: **true**   **false**

12. Most people with unipolar disorder experience only a single, isolated episode during their lifetimes: **true**   **false**

13. People with Bipolar I Disorder have clear cut _____ episodes, while people with Bipolar II Disorder do not.

14. Rapid cycling bipolar patients typically do not respond as well to treatment as other bipolar patients: **true**   **false**

15. People with seasonal depression are more likely to gain weight and sleep more than people with nonseasonal depression patterns: **true**   **false**

16. The average age of onset of a first episode of unipolar disorder is at which age:
    adolescence (15-25)   **young adulthood (25-35)**   **middle age (40-50)**

17. The average number of lifetime depressive episodes of people with unipolar disorder is _____.

18. A person's risk of _____ of depression goes down the longer they are in remission.

19. The average age of onset of a first episode of bipolar disorder is at which age:

    adolescence (15-25)   young adulthood (25-35)   middle age (40-50)

20. People with bipolar disorder tend to have more episodes than those with unipolar disorder: **true   false**

21. According to the Cross-National Collaborative Study, lifetime risk for major depressive disorder is _____%; for dysthymia is _____%; and for bipolar disorder is _____%.

22. Many, even most, people with mood disorders do not seek treatment:

    true   false

23. What sex is more likely to experience major depression and dysthymia? _____

24. There are no significant gender differences in rates of _____.

25. Some studies indicate similar frequencies of mood disorders in different countries and cultures, but differences in specific symptoms. For example, depressed people in Europe and North America are more likely to exhibit _____ while depressed people in non-Western countries, like China, are more likely to exhibit _____.

26. Mood disorders are less common among the elderly than among young and middle-aged adults: **true   false**

27. The frequency of depression has decreased in recent years: **true   false**

28. Prospective research design has demonstrated that which one comes first, depression or stressful events? _____

29. Research has shown that the _____ of an important person or role precipitates depression.

30. Once a person is depressed, their behaviour does lead to an increase in their levels of stress: **true   false**

31. Bipolar patients who leave the hospital to live with hostile, critical family members are more likely to experience _____.

32. Research indicates that communities with the highest rates of severe events have the highest prevalence of _____.

33. Beck described several types of cognitive distortions he thought were related to depression. Research has shown that these distortions are present during an episode of depression but not before or after an episode: **true**   **false**

34. A depressogenic attributional style is characterized by a tendency to explain negative events, like failing an exam, in which of the following terms:
    external or **internal**;   **stable** or **unstable**;   **specific** or **global**

35. College students who had negative cognitive styles at the beginning of freshman year were much more likely to develop _____.

36. Lewinsohn hypothesized that some depressed behaviours may initially be reinforced by friends and family and the strength and frequency of these behaviours are:
    increased   **decreased**

37. Coyne hypothesized that depressed people actually do have smaller and less supportive social networks, and that it is not just their perceptions but the actual situation that is negative. Does the research evidence support this? _____

38. People with a ruminative style have   **more** or **less**   depression that people with a distracting style. Men are **more** or **less** likely to have a ruminative style than women.

39. Among relatives of people with unipolar disorder, there **is** or **is not** an increased risk for unipolar disorder, and there   **is** or **is not** an increased risk for bipolar disorder.

40. Which disorder, major depressive disorder, bipolar disorder, or dysthymia, shows the highest rate of twin concordance (genetic heritability)? _____ Which shows the lowest? _____

41. Researchers think that the genetic influence on mood disorders is due to:
    a single gene   **multiple genes**

42. Current research on the role of neurotransmitters in the aetiology of depression suggests that the early theories (the catecholamine hypothesis and the indolamine hypothesis) were too complex: **true**   **false**

43. There are approximately **3 50 100** different neurotransmitters in the central nervous system.

44. Brain imaging studies have failed to find any differences in brain function related to mood: **true   false**

45. Rats exposed to stressful events in the laboratory develop symptoms similar to those of depressed people, and antidepressant drugs given to these animals can reverse or prevent these symptoms: **true   false**

46. In treating depressed people, _____ therapy focuses on changing the client's negative schemas and irrational beliefs, and _____ therapy focuses on changing current relationships.

47. Antidepressants typically are effective within 24 hours if they are going to be helpful at all: **true   false**

48. Antidepressant medication is far more effective in treating depression than either cognitive or interpersonal therapy: **true   false**

49. Among patients with seasonal affective disorder, exposure to broad-spectrum light is actually *not* effective in reducing depression: **true   false**

50. ECT almost always interferes with memory: **true   false**

51. What percentage of people with mood disorders will eventually commit suicide?
    1-3%   15-20%   50-55%

52. Suicide is increasing among adolescents in recent decades: **true   false**

53. There are gender differences in rates of suicide: more **males** or **females** make suicide attempts, and more   **males** or **females** actually complete a suicide.

54. Which group has the highest rate of suicide:
    young black men,   middle-aged white women,   older white men?

55. Does suicide run in families? _____

56. Media coverage of a suicide increases the rate of suicides committed: **true false**

57. Suicide hotlines decrease suicide rates: **true   false**

Multiple Choice Questions

The following multiple choice questions will test your comprehension of the material presented in the chapter. Answers are listed at the end of the chapter.

1) Which of the following is NOT a general area describing the signs and symptoms representative of mood disorders?

   a. emotional symptoms
   b. psychological symptoms

   c. somatic symptoms
   d. cognitive symptoms

2) A promising form of treatment for seasonal affective disorder is:

   a. light therapy
   b. lithium carbonate

   c. nutritional therapy
   d. meditation

3) What is the percent of completed suicides that occur as a result of a primary mood disorder?

   a. under 15%
   b. under 30%

   c. over 50%
   d. over 78%

4) Which is an example of a somatic symptom?

   a. suicidal ideation
   b. loss of interest

   c. sleep disturbance
   d. low self-esteem

5) An advantage of an analogue study is that:

   a. experimental procedures may be employed
   b. it is easy to generalize the results beyond the laboratory
   c. human subjects are not used
   d. it is easy to reproduce a clinical disorder in the laboratory

6) Which symptom would NOT be considered diagnostic for clinical depression?

   a. racing thoughts
   b. fatigue or loss of energy

   c. feelings of worthlessness
   d. difficulty concentrating

7) Why might it be more difficult to diagnose depression in the elderly?

   a. cognitive impairment or other problems common in the elderly may mask the symptoms of depression
   b. the elderly are more reluctant to seek treatment for depression
   c. the symptoms and features of depression change as age increases
   d. the elderly are less likely to report somatic symptoms associated with depression

8) Results from the Treatment of Depression Collaborative Research Program indicate that:

   a. both types of psychological treatment (interpersonal and cognitive) were as effective as antidepressant medication
   b. patients who received interpersonal therapy did not show gains with cognitive problems
   c. placebo was equally effective to antidepressant medication
   d. cognitive therapy was superior to interpersonal therapy in its effectiveness

9) Which age group has experienced increased rates of suicide since the 1960s?

   a. adolescents
   b. people who are in their 30's
   c. people between the ages of 45 and 55
   d. people over 65

10) When two loci occupy positions close together on the same chromosome they are:

   a. polygenic
   b. matched
   c. homogenous
   d. linked

11) Which is a social factor which may contribute to the onset of depression?

   a. the belief that one cannot control events in one's life
   b. cognitive distortions
   c. stressful life events
   d. neuroendocrine disturbances

12) Which disorder is often comorbid with a mood disorder?

   a. schizophrenia
   b. dissociative disorder
   c. paranoid personality disorder
   d. alcoholism

13) What age would a person most likely have a first episode of bipolar disorder?

   a. 18 – 23 years
   b. 28 – 33 years
   c. 38 – 43 years
   d. 48 – 53 years

14) Which of the following is a common element of suicide?

   a. the common goal of suicide is cessation of consciousness
   b. the common emotion in suicide is anger
   c. the common purpose of suicide is to get revenge
   d. the common stressor in suicide is financial difficulties

15) Decreased need for sleep, pressure to keep talking, grandiosity, and distractibility are common symptoms of which disorder?

   a. mania
   b. dysthymia
   c. major depression
   d. cyclothymia

16) Advantages of selective serotonin reuptake inhibitors include all EXCEPT:

   a. fewer side effects
   b. less likely to have multiple episodes of depression
   c. less dangerous in the case of an overdose
   d. easier for the patient to take

17) Which is an example of a depressogenic premise?

   a. "I find time in my day to relax"
   b. "I should be at the top of my performance at all times"
   c. "I congratulate myself when I finish a hard day at work"
   d. "I try to forgive myself when I screw things up"

18) Research on electroconvulsive therapy supports that:

   a. memory impairment may be permanent
   b. only bipolar depressed patients respond to ECT
   c. ECT is as effective as placebo
   d. some depressed patients may respond to ECT more than to antidepressants

19) Which statement is NOT true about unipolar depression?

   a. episodes of unipolar depression tend to be longer in duration, compared to episodes of depression in bipolar disorder
   b. at least half of unipolar patients will experience more than one episode
   c. female patients tend to relapse more quickly than male patients
   d. unipolar patients have their first episode at a much younger age than do bipolar patients

20) Some depressed people exhibit a depressogenic attributional style that is characterized by the tendency to explain negative events in terms of:

   a. internal, stable, global factors
   b. internal, unstable, specific factors
   c. external, unstable, specific factors
   d. external, stable, specific factors

21) A standard part of cognitive treatment for depression would be:

   a. gaining insight into suppressed anger in close relationships
   b. developing a better understanding of family relationships
   c. substituting more flexible self-statements for rigid and absolute ones
   d. nondirect discussions of unexpressed emotions

22) An important assumption of the hopelessness theory of depression is:

    a. loss of a parent early in life increases risk for depression
    b. desirable events will not occur regardless of what the person does
    c. depressed people are more likely to feel in control of the events of their lives
    d. depressed people have a positive impact on other people's moods

23) Which type of coping behaviour is associated with longer and more severely depressed moods?

    a. processing style   c. intellectual style
    b. ruminative style   d. distracting style

24) Studies investigating genetic transmission of mood disorders indicate that:

    a. genetic factors are more influential in bipolar disorders than major depressive disorder
    b. the concordance rate for mood disorders is higher for DZ than MZ twins
    c. there is no increased risk of bipolar disorder for relatives of bipolar patients
    d. genetic factors account for about 90% of the variance for dysthymia

25) How do depressed people often respond to a test dose of dexamethasone?

    a. they show a suppression of cortisol secretion
    b. they show a failure of suppression of cortisol secretion
    c. they show a dramatic increase of cortisol secretion
    d. they show an abnormal fluctuation of cortisol secretion

26) An example of DSM-IV subtype of depression is:

    a. retarded   c. narcissistic
    b. dysphoric   d. melancholic

27) Which of the following areas of the brain have not been found to show changes in activity when mood is disturbed?

    a. cerebellum   c. hypothalamus
    b. amydala   d. limbic system

Understanding Research — Fill in the Blank

Social Origins of Depression in Women: The text presents in detailed description of a study by Brown, Bifulco, and Harris in the Research Close-Up. Finding the answers to these questions will help you get a good understanding of this study and why it is important. It is not necessary to memorize the answers; the process of finding them in the textbook will help you learn the material you need to know.

1. Did men or women participate? _____ Ages of subjects were from
   _____ to _____. Why did all subjects selected have children living at
   home? _____

   _____

2. What information did they gather for each subject? Psychological adjustment (like
   symptoms of _____ _____ and self-_____).
   Living circumstances (like _____ relationships and social _____).

3. At follow-up one year later, they asked about _____ events and difficulties
   of the previous year, and they asked again about _____ of mental
   disorders. Judges rating each description of life events could use all information for
   making ratings but _____ and

   _____.

4. How many women were NOT depressed at Time I? _____ What percent
   of women who did not experience a severe event during the follow up year became
   depressed? _____% What percent of women who became depressed had
   experienced a severe event prior to becoming depressed? _____% What
   does this show are associated? _____

5. Only 3% of women experiencing a severe event involving _____ became
   depressed, but almost _____% of those did when the event was considered
   _____. Also, feeling of _____ made a woman three times more
   likely to become depressed.

6. Why is the use of a prospective design important here? _____
   _____. What is the direction of effect
   indicated by these findings? _____ cause(s) _____.

Analogue Studies of Psychopathology: The text discusses this type of research in the
Research Methods section. Finding the answers to these questions will help you get a
good understanding of this research method.

7. What is the key difference between a correlational study and an experiment?

   _____

   _____

8. Why can't researchers do experiments about the causes of psychopathology with human subjects? _____

_____

9. Harlow's research showed that rhesus monkey infants separated from their mothers showed symptoms similar to symptoms of _____in people. What can protect these infant monkeys from the detrimental effects of maternal separation?

_____

_____

10. What is one criticism of analogue models of depression? _____

_____

_____

11. Not all analogue studies use animals. The Little Albert study involved a human infant repeatedly exposed to the pairing of a white _____ with a loud, startling noise. The infant's behaviour was seen as an analogue of clinical _____. What is a criticism of analogue studies in general?

_____

Brief Essay

As a final exercise, write out answers to the following brief essay questions. Then compare your answers with the material presented in the text.

After you have answered these questions, review the "critical thinking" questions that are presented at the end of the text chapter. Answering these questions will help you integrate important issues and themes that have been featured throughout the chapter.

1. What primary issues have been at the centre of the controversy about mood disorder definitions? Would you advocate the use of subtyping? Why?

2. Discuss the methodological problems that one encounters in studying mood disorder across cultures. How have cross-cultural investigations assisted our understanding of mood disorders?

3. Describe the model of depression that emphasizes the interplay between cognitive and interpersonal factors.

ANSWER KEY

Key Terms — Matching #1

1. u	9. n	17. e
2. m	10. t	18. k
3. d	11. a	19. f
4. v	12. h	20. l
5. q	13. s	21. r
6. b	14. c	22. o
7. p	15. i	
8. g	16. j	

Names You Should Know

1. a
2. c
3. d
4. b
5. e
6. f

Key Terms — Matching #2

a. 11	d. 6	g. 3	j. 9	m. 10	p. 5
b. 7	e. 4	h. 15	k. 16	n. 14
c. 13	f. 1	i. 8	l. 2	o. 12

Review of Concepts

1. true
2. true
3. concentrating, decisions
4. themselves, their environment, the future
5. mania
6. depression
7. false
8. false
9. depression; mania
10. alcoholism, eating disorders, anxiety disorders
11. true
12. false
13. manic
14. true
15. true
16. middle age
17. 5 or 6
18. relapse
19. young adulthood
20. true
21. 10%; 0.6%; 6%
22. true
23. females
24. bipolar disorder
25. guilt and suicidal feelings; somatic feelings
26. true
27. false
28. stressful event
29. loss
30. true
31. relapse
32. depression
33. true
34. internal, stable, global
35. major depressive disorder
36. increased
37. yes
38. more; less
39. is; is not
40. bipolar disorder, dysthymia
41. multiple genes
42. false
43. 100

44. false
45. true
46. cognitive, interpersonal
47. false
48. false
49. false
50. false
51. 15-20%

52. true
53. females, males
54. older white men
55. yes
56. true
57. false

Multiple Choice

1. b	6. a	11. c	16. b	21. c	26. d
2. a	7. a	12. d	17. b	22. b	27. a
3. c	8. a	13. b	18. d	23. b	
4. c	9. a	14. a	19. d	24. a	
5. a	10. d	15. a	20. a	25. a	

Understanding Research

1. women; 18 to 50; because they found that women with children at home are more likely to become depressed

2. mental disorders; esteem; personal; support

3. life; symptoms; the woman's mental status; how she responded to the stressful event

4. 303; 2; 90; stressful life events and depression

5. danger; 40; humiliating; entrapment

6. It shows that the depression follows the stressful life event; stressful life events cause depression

7. You can't make a case that one thing causes another in a correlational study but you can in an experiment.

8. It is unethical to attempt to cause psychopathology in people.

9. depression; lots of experience with peers and adult monkeys other than the mother

10. Cognitive symptoms of depression can't be measured in (and may not be experienced by) animals

11. rat; phobia; Results in an artificial laboratory situation may not be generalisable to the real world.

CHAPTER 6
ANXIETY DISORDERS

Chapter Outline

I. Overview

II. Typical Symptoms and Associated Features
    A. Anxiety
    B. Excessive Worry
    C. Panic Attacks
    D. Phobias
    E. Obsessions and Compulsions

III. Classification
    A. Brief Historical Perspective
    B. Contemporary Diagnostic Systems
    C. Subclassification
    D. Course and Outcome

IV. Epidemiology
    A. Prevalence
    B. Comorbidity
    C. Gender Differences
    D. Anxiety Across the Life Span
    E. Cross-Cultural Comparisons

V. Aetiological Considerations and Research
    A. Social Factors
        1. Stressful Life Events
        2. Childhood Adversity
        3. Attachment Relationships and Separation Anxiety
    B. Psychological Factors
        1. Learning Processes and Phobias
            a. Preparedness
            b. Observational Learning
        2. Cognitive Factors
            a. Perception of Control
            b. Catastrophic Misinterpretation
            c. Attention to Threat and Shifts in Attention
            d. Thought Suppression: Obsessive-Compulsive Disorder
    C. Biological Factors
        1. Genetic Factors
            a. Family Studies
            b. Twin Studies

2. Neurochemistry
3. False Suffocation Alarms: An Integrated Systems Model

VI. Treatment
    A. Psychological Interventions
       1. Systematic Desensitisation and Interoceptive Exposure
       2. Exposure and Response Prevention
       3. Relaxation and Breathing Retraining
       4. Cognitive Therapy
    B. Biological Interventions
       1. Antianxiety Medications
       2. Antidepressant Medications

Learning Objectives

After reviewing the material presented in this chapter, you should be able to:

1. Contrast anxiety with fear; define anxiety and worry.

2. Name some of the key physical and cognitive symptoms in panic attacks

3. Compare specific phobias with agoraphobia

4. Define obsessions and compulsions

5. Understand the Freudian theory of anxiety.

6. Know the basic classification system that DSM-IV uses for panic disorder, specific phobia, social phobia, generalised anxiety disorder, obsessive-compulsive disorder, and agoraphobia.

7. Rank the prevalence rates of anxiety disorders in order.

8. Understand the role of evolution in anxiety and anxiety disorders.

9. Recognise the role of social factors (stressful life events and childhood adversity) in the development of anxiety disorders.

10. Understand the way in which Seligman's preparedness model helps to explain why certain phobias are "easier"(fear-relevant) to develop.

11. Name four cognitive factors that are considered influential in the development of anxiety disorders.

12. Describe the results of family studies and twin studies of incidence of anxiety disorders.

13. Recognise the role of neurochemistry in anxiety disorders.

14. Appreciate the differences between systematic desensitisation and flooding in treatment of phobias.

15. Describe how cognitive therapy is used in the treatment of anxiety disorders.

16. Know the advantages and disadvantages of using benzodiazepines and tricyclics in the treatment of various anxiety disorders.

Key Terms — Matching #1

The following terms related to anxiety disorders are important to know. To test your knowledge, match the following terms with their definitions. Answers are listed at the end of the chapter.

a. Fear
b. Anxiety
c. Worry
d. Panic attack
e. Phobia
f. Agoraphobia

g. Social phobia
h. Specific phobia
i. Preparedness
j. Observational learning
k. Experimental neurosis

1. ____ induced in laboratory animals under stressful performance requirements, such as making extremely difficult discriminations; characterised by anxiety and agitation, increased startle responses, and disruption of feeding
2. ____ a sudden, overwhelming experience of focused terror
3. ____ an emotion experienced in the face of real, immediate danger
4. ____ phobia of public spaces, or fear of not being able to escape or of having a panic attack in such places
5. ____ phobia cued by doing something, such as speaking or eating, in front of other people who might scrutinise the performance
6. ____ an emotional reaction out of proportion to threats from the environment
7. ____ a phobia cued by the presence of a specific object or situation
8. ____ persistent, irrational fears associated with a specific object or situation that lead the person to avoid the feared stimulus
9. ____ proposes that organisms are biologically predisposed, on the basis of neural pathways, to learn certain types of associations more quickly
10. ____ a more or less uncontrollable sequence of negative, emotional thoughts and images concerned with possible future danger
11. ____ learning behaviours through imitation of a model

Key Terms — Matching #2

The following terms related to anxiety disorders are important to know. To test your knowledge, match the following terms with their definitions. Answers are listed at the end of the chapter.

1. Obsessions
2. Compulsions
3. Neurosis
4. Signal anxiety
5. Generalised anxiety disorder
6. Catastrophic misinterpretation
7. Situational exposure
8. Interoceptive exposure

9. Thought suppression
10. Pharmacological challenge procedures
11. False suffocation alarm
12. Flooding
13. Benzodiazepines
14. Azapirones
15. Breathing retraining

a. _____ indicates that an instinctual impulse previously associated with punishment and disapproval is about to be acted upon

b. _____ exposure beginning with the most frightening stimuli

c. _____ repetitive, unwanted, intrusive thoughts, images, or impulses

d. _____ minor tranquilizers frequently used in the treatment of anxiety disorders

e. _____ an active attempt to stop thinking about something that often leads to the paradoxical effect of an increase in strong emotions associated with unpleasant thoughts

f. _____ repetitive, ritualistic behaviour aimed at reducing anxiety; the person perceives it as irrational and tries to resist performing it but cannot

g. _____ a disorder characterised by excessive and uncontrollable worry about a number of events or activities and associated symptoms of arousal

h. _____ a misfire of the system that detects carbon dioxide, which can also be set off by lactate infusion; may cause panic attacks

i. _____ a psychoanalytic term describing persistent emotional disturbances, such as anxiety or depression, in which anxiety is the key characteristic

j. _____ perceiving bodily sensations as a signal of an impending disastrous event, such as a heart attack

k. _____ a research procedure where a particular brain mechanism is stressed by the artificial administration of chemicals, which if it leads to a panic attack may implicate that brain mechanism in the aetiology of panic attack

l. _____ a treatment for agoraphobia which involves repeatedly confronting the situation that has previously been avoided

m. _____ learning to take slow deep breaths

n. _____ a treatment for panic disorder which involves standardised exercises that produce sensations often felt during a panic attack

o. _____ antianxiety medications which act on serotonin transmission

Names You Should Know — Matching

The following people have played an important role in research and theory of anxiety disorders. To test your knowledge, match the following names with the descriptions of their contributions to the study of abnormal psychology. Answers are listed at the end of the chapter.

a. Susan Mineka
b. David Clark
c. Sigmund Freud
d. Thomas Borkovec

e. John Bowlby
f. Kenneth Kendler
g. Martin Seligman
h. S.J. Rachman

1. _____ studied the influence of genes and environment on anxiety disorders; found that their influences are fairly disorder-specific
2. _____ conducted a series of studies with rhesus monkeys that combined observational learning with preparedness theory
3. _____ proposed preparedness theory, that people are prepared to develop intense, persistent fears to certain stimuli
4. _____ developed a theory of anxiety based on work with many patients; sees anxiety as warning the person they are about to do or think something that is unacceptable and triggering ego defences to prevent the thought or action
5. _____ saw anxiety as an innate response to separation or threat of separation from caregiver
6. _____ conducted research on catastrophic misinterpretation
7. _____ researched uncontrollable worry; conceptualised it as a verbal rather than visual event which distracts the person from imagery that would trigger unpleasant somatic arousal
8. _____ researched how normal people respond to traumatic and threatening situations

Review of Concepts — Fill in the Blank and True/False

This section will help focus your studying by testing whether you understand the concepts presented in the text. After you have read and reviewed the material, test your comprehension and memory by filling in the following blanks or circling the right answer. Answers are listed at the end of the chapter.

1. There is a lot of overlap between anxiety disorders and depression:

      true   false

2. Maladaptive anxiety, or anxious apprehension, consists of:

      1) _____,

      2) _____, and

      3) _____.

3. Panic attacks have what type of onset: **gradual   sudden**

4. Panic attacks can happen when the person is in bed: **true   false**

5. Agoraphobia is different from other phobias in that agoraphobics are often afraid they will lose _____ in public.

6. List two ways that obsessions are different from worry; obsessions:

   1) _____, and

   2) _____.

7. Normal people seldom experience obsessions: **true   false**

8. Which is a common compulsion?   **scratching   coughing   cleaning**

9. People with anxiety disorders typically require hospitalization: **true   false**

10. The Freudian explanation of obsessive-compulsive disorder is that the patient has serious difficulties in dealing with what emotion? _____

11. Experts who classify mental disorders can be described as "lumpers" or "splitters;" earlier classification systems used the lumping or splitting approach and contemporary systems use the lumping or splitting approach.

12. Intrusive thoughts about real problems are one form of obsessions:

    true   false

13. Panic disorder usually goes away without treatment: **true   false**

14. Many patients with obsessive-compulsive disorder show improved levels of functioning over time although they may continue to have some symptoms:

    true   false

15. Anxiety disorders are the most common form of mental disorder: **true   false**

16. What percent of people who meet the criteria for one anxiety disorder also meet the criteria for another anxiety disorder?   **5%   20%   50%**

17. Anxiety and depression are closely related concepts, but Clark and Watson have proposed a model using positive and negative affect to help distinguish between them. Anxiety and depression both share high negative affect, but anxiety alone is

characterised by _____ and depression alone is characterised

by _____.

18. Depressive disorders and anxiety disorders show high comorbidity; another disorder with high comorbidity with anxiety disorders is_____.

19. People with an anxiety disorder have a greater risk of developing alcohol dependence: **true**   **false**

20. Which are more likely to experience specific phobias?   **men**   **women**

21. Which anxiety disorder occurs equally frequently among men and women?

_____

22. What percentage of people with agoraphobia also report symptoms of panic disorder?   **20%**   **50%**   **95%**

23. What age group has the lowest prevalence of anxiety disorders?_____

24. Anxiety disorders are almost entirely specific to people in Western societies: very few people in nonindustrialised countries experience them: **true**   **false**

25. Stressful life events have been linked to both depressive disorders and anxiety disorders. In one study, women who experienced an event involving _____were more likely to experience depression and those who experienced an event involving _____ were more likely to experience anxiety.

26. What personality factors are associated with elevated risk for panic attacks?

_____

27. Two types of childhood adversity were linked to adult anxiety disorders, especially panic disorder; they were_____ and

_____ ; specific phobia was unrelated to childhood adversity.

28. People who have agoraphobia were more likely to have had an _____ attachment to their parents as toddlers.

29. Seligman identified several shortcomings with the classical conditioning model of phobias. They are 1) Conditioned fear responses learned in a laboratory are easy to _____, while phobic responses are extremely persistent;

2) Phobias developed after traumatic experiences, in contrast to those learned in the laboratory, are developed after _____ trial, and 3) The theory states that any stimulus can be conditioned to provoke fear, but phobias of guns, cars, and electrical outlets, potentially dangerous objects, are_____.

30. Monitoring one's heart rate when aroused minimises the fear response:
    true   false

31. Rhesus monkeys raised in the wild   **are**   or   **are not**   afraid of snakes, while those raised in a laboratory   **are**   or   **are not**   afraid of snakes.

32. Monkeys can learn to fear snakes by watching videotapes of other monkeys exhibiting fear reactions toward snakes: **true   false**

33. People who believe they are able to control their environment are   **more   or   less** likely to show symptoms of anxiety than people who believe they are helpless.

34. One piece of evidence of the limitations of the catastrophic misinterpretation model of panic attacks is that they can occur while a person is _____.

35. In contrast to a depressed person, who is convinced that failure will occur, an anxious person is _____ that failure will occur.

36 Thought suppression has been found to be quite effective in reducing worrying and intrusive thoughts: **true   false**

37. Relatives of people with panic disorder are more likely to have panic disorder but not more likely to have generalised anxiety disorder: **true   false**

38. Relatives of people with generalised anxiety disorder are more likely to have GAD but not more likely to have panic disorder: **true   false**

39. Relatives of people with obsessive-compulsive disorder are more likely to have OCD but not more likely to have other anxiety disorders: **true   false**

40. There is no evidence that the findings that anxiety disorders run in families can be explained in part by genetic influences: **true   false**

41. Injecting anxiety disorder patients with lactate almost always triggered a panic attack, while only a few control subjects experienced one: **true   false**

42. Which of the following substances can trigger panic attack in anxiety patients?

    alcohol   caffeine   aspirin

43. Exposure to the feared object, situation, or behaviour is an effective treatment for anxiety disorders: **true   false**

44. The best form of behaviour therapy for OCD is _____.

45. Cognitive therapy for anxiety disorders often involves analyzing errors in the patient's _____ as well as the process of _____.

46. Antianxiety medications are particularly effective in reducing a person's worry and rumination: **true   false**

47. Benzodiazepines are more effective in the treatment of _____ and _____ and less effective in the treatment of _____ and _____.

48. Benzodiazepines are addictive: **true   false**

49. Antidepressants are effective in treating some anxiety disorders: **true   false**

50. Mixed Anxiety-Depressive Disorder is an official DSM-IV-TR Anxiety Disorder which is characterised by the co-occurrence of severe anxiety and depression.

    true   false

Multiple Choice Questions

The following multiple choice questions will test your comprehension of the material presented in the chapter. Answers are listed at the end of the chapter.

1) The most frequently used types of minor tranquilizers for the treatment of anxiety disorders are:

    a. tricyclics
    b. benzodiazapines
    c. serotonin
    d. GABA inhibitors

2) Which of the following is LEAST likely to be present in an anxiety disorder?

    a. lack of insight
    b. social impairment
    c. significant personal distress
    d. negative emotional response

3) Which of the following is an example of a potential unconditioned stimulus (UCS) which could contribute to the development of a phobia?

   a. loss of a relationship
   b. chronic occupational difficulties
   c. a painfully loud and unexpected noise
   d. a sad song

4) _____ is experienced in the face of real, immediate danger, _____ is a diffuse reaction that is out of proportion to threats from the environment.

   a. anxiety, fear   c. fear, anxiety
   b. worry, anxiety   d. worry, fear

5) Results of family studies investigating transmission of anxiety disorders suggest:

   a. there appears to be no genetic component to OCD
   b. social phobia is the most inheritable form of anxiety disorder
   c. panic disorder and GAD are etiologically separate disorders
   d. the most inheritable anxiety disorder is specific phobia

6) The two most common types of compulsions are:

   a. counting and repeating   c. sorting and counting
   b. cleaning and checking   d. checking and writing

7) A junior in college, Sam is acutely distressed at the thought of having to write in front of others. He is afraid that he will drop his pen, lose control of his writing, or somehow embarrass himself while other people are watching. He is able to write when alone, but this fear has impaired his ability to take notes in class. His diagnosis would be:

   a. specific phobia   c. generalised anxiety disorder
   b. agoraphobia   d. social phobia

8) The discovery of laboratory procedures that reliably induce panic attacks is important because:

   a. they offer investigators the opportunity to research the antecedents and consequences of panic attacks
   b. brain activities that occur during a panic attack may be monitored
   c. such procedures may be fruitful in developing a map of the specific areas of the brain that mediate anxiety symptoms
   d. all of the above

9) Which of the following is the most common type of abnormal behaviour?

   a. phobias   c. generalised anxiety disorder
   b. major depression   d. dysthymia

10) Specific phobias may be best understood in terms of learning experiences. The association between the object and intense fear can develop through all BUT which of the following?

    a. direct experience
    b. observational learning
    c. exposure to fear-irrelevant stimuli
    d. exposure to warnings about dangerous situations

11) Which is TRUE regarding the relationship between anxiety and other disorders?

    a. substance dependence is rarely associated with anxiety disorders
    b. anxiety disorders overlap considerably with other anxiety disorders
    c. anxiety disorders usually overlap with psychotic disorders
    d. anxiety disorders do not appear to be associated with depressive disorders

12) "Free-floating" anxiety would be most characteristic of which anxiety disorder?

    a. social phobia
    b. panic disorder
    c. obsessive-compulsive disorder
    d. generalised anxiety disorder

13) Which of the following is NOT consistent with Freud's model of anxiety?

    a. repression is the product of anxiety
    b. anxiety is the result of a harsh superego in conflict with the defence mechanisms that are employed by the ego
    c. the specific form of overt symptoms is determined by the defence mechanisms that are employed by the ego
    d. different types of anxiety disorders can be distinguished by many factors within the analytic framework, for example, the developmental stage at which the person experiences problems

14) Anxiety disorder categories did not emerge in psychiatric classifications during the last century primarily because:

    a. the prevalence of anxiety disorders was much lower during the last century
    b. they were considered to be neurological disorders
    c. very few cases of anxiety disorders required institutionalisation
    d. physicians were not trained to recognise the symptoms of anxiety disorders

15) Which of the following is NOT a symptom of a panic attack?

    a. feeling of choking
    b. trembling
    c. nausea
    d. headache

16) Research on the relationship between stressful life events and anxiety disorders suggests that:

    a. the onset of agoraphobia may be associated with interpersonal conflict
    b. marital distress is associated with the onset of simple phobia

c. the onset of agoraphobia may be associated with the experience of a conditioning event, such as a sudden painful injury

d. severe loss is associated with the onset of an anxiety disorder

17) Which cognitive factor shares an important relationship with panic attacks?

a. perception of control over events in one's environment
b. thought suppression
c. cognitive minimisation of traumatic events
d. all-or-none thinking about future events

18) Which is NOT included in the DSM-IV's classification of anxiety disorders?

a. panic disorder
b. agoraphobia
c. cyclothymia
d. obsessive-compulsive disorder

19) If a panic attack only occurs in the presence of a particular stimulus, it is said to be:

a. a situationally cued attack
b. an anticipated attack
c. a "below threshold" attack
d. a cognitively processed attack

20) Karen has consistent worries that she is going to lose her job, that something is going to happen to her husband and that she will be alone, and that her health may take a turn for the worse. She knows that her worries are causing friction in her marriage, but she feels that she cannot control them, although she repeatedly tries to put them out of her mind. Although she has always been a "worrier", the intensity and frequency of her worries has worsened in the past year. Her diagnosis would be:

a. agoraphobia
b. panic disorder
c. generalised anxiety disorder
d. simple phobia

21) The most serious adverse side effects of benzodiazepines is:

a. heart palpitations
b. significant weight gain
c. necessary dietary restrictions
d. their potential for addiction

22) The types of symptoms most characteristic of a panic attack are:

a. interpersonal difficulties
b. physical sensations
c. emotional reactions
d. cognitive reactions

23) Cross-cultural research on anxiety disorders suggests that:

a. anxiety disorders are not experienced in certain cultures
b. phobic avoidance is the most commonly reported symptom across cultures
c. the focus of typical anxiety complaints can vary dramatically across cultures
d. anxiety disorders are more common in preliterate cultures

24) An important consideration in diagnosing panic disorder is that the person must:

    a. experience recurrent, situationally cued panic attacks
    b. experience recurrent panic attacks in anticipation of a feared event
    c. report the experience of feeling out of control
    d. experience recurrent unexpected panic attacks

25) Which of the following is NOT included in the DSM-IV as criteria to establish the boundary between normal behaviour and compulsive rituals?

    a. the rituals cause marked distress
    b. the rituals can be observed by other people
    c. the rituals interfere with normal occupational and social functioning
    d. the rituals take more than one hour per day to perform

26) Which of the following would be a typical situation that would cause problems for an agoraphobic?

    a. travelling on the subway   c. cleaning the house
    b. speaking to a friend on the phone   d. encountering a snake

27) According to recent research, what percent of the people who qualify for an anxiety disorder diagnosis actually seek treatment for their disorder?

    a. 15%   c. 40%
    b. 25%   d. 50%

28) What is an important difference between compulsions and some addictive behaviours such as gambling?

    a. addictive behaviours reduce anxiety more effectively than compulsions
    b. compulsions are more resistant to treatment
    c. addictive behaviours are not repetitive in nature
    d. compulsions reduce anxiety but they do not produce pleasure

29) Women are at least twice as likely as men to experience all BUT which of the following anxiety disorders?

    a. obsessive-compulsive disorder   c. specific phobia
    b. agoraphobia   d. panic disorder

Understanding Research — Fill in the Blank

Panic and Perception of Control: The text presents a detailed description of a study by Sanderson, Rapee, and Barlow in the Research Close-Up. Finding the answers to these questions will help you get a good understanding of this study and why it is important. It is not necessary to memorise the answers; the process of finding them in the textbook will help you learn the material you need to know.

1. All of the procedures researchers have used to induce a panic attack in a laboratory situation produce a range of peripheral _____ sensations, such as _____, chest _____, and _____- headedness.

2. In this study they used air enriched with _____ but manipulated the subjects' impressions of whether they were in _____ of the air mixture. All subjects met diagnostic criteria for _____ disorder.

3. Each person sat _____in a quiet room, breathing through a gas ____, and rated his or her _____level. They were told when the box was _____ they could adjust the mixture of carbon dioxide by using the dial on their _____. In reality the dial had _____effect. All patients received _____ minutes of compressed air, then _____ minutes of carbon-dioxide enriched air. For ____ of the _____ patients the light went on, and for the rest it never went on.

4. Following the procedure, subjects were all interviewed to see if they experienced a _____. Eight of the 10 subjects in the _____ group had a panic attack. Two of the 10 subjects in the _____ group had a panic attack. Those in the no illusion group reported more than _____ as many symptoms than those in the illusion of control group. Both groups had symptoms of breathlessness and _____ sensations, dizziness, _____ heatedness, and pounding _____.

5. This study is important because it shows how biological and psychological factors _____ to produce the experience of panic. Biological factors were important but alone were not _____ to produce an attack. Feelings of _____ were particularly important.

Statistical Significance and Clinical Importance: The text discusses this type of research in the Research Methods section. Finding the answers to these questions will help you get a good understanding of these issues.

6. Does a statistical difference always mean the finding is clinically significant? _____ What disorder is used in the hypothetical example? _____ What is the null hypothesis? _____ What is the other hypothesis? _____

_____

7. Statistically significant tests are ones where the probability of finding the difference that you are observing among the groups by chance alone is less than _____ times out of 100. In the hypothesised study, outcome was rated on a scale of anxiety ranging from _____ to _____. Both groups had a mean rating of _____ prior to treatment, and after treatment the difference between the two treatment groups was _____ points.

8. Why is this difference not clinically important? _____

_____

_____

Brief Essay

As a final exercise, write out answers to the following brief essay questions. Then compare your answers with the material presented in the text.

After you have answered these questions, review the "critical thinking" questions that are presented at the end of the text chapter. Answering these questions will help you integrate important issues and themes that have been featured throughout the chapter.

1. Learning processes have been theoretically associated with the development of phobias, while cognitive factors have been used to explain the development of panic attacks. Review the prominent learning and cognitive theories that account for each type of disorder. Do you think that differences in etiological processes imply that these disorders are really unrelated? Why or why not?

2. Discuss the overlap between anxiety and depression. Do you think that anxiety and depression are separate types of disorders, or do you think that they represent different manifestations of the same problem? What evidence supports your position?

3. Consider the following psychological interventions used for the treatment of anxiety disorders: desensitisation, flooding, prolonged exposure and response prevention, and cognitive therapy. Select an anxiety disorder and discuss how you would approach treatment for this disorder. Which intervention techniques(s) would you choose and why?

4. False suffocation alarm theory is a theoretical model of panic attacks and agoraphobia that integrates biological and psychological factors. Discuss this theory, highlighting both the main assumptions of the model and the research findings which support these assumptions.

ANSWER KEY

Key Terms — Matching #1

1. k	5. g	9. i
2. d	6. b	10. c
3. a	7. h	11. j
4. f	8. e	

Names You Should Know

1. f	5. e
2. a	6. b
3. g	7. d
4. c	8. h

Key Terms — Matching #2

a. 4	d. 13	g. 5	j. 6	m. 15
b. 12	e. 9	h. 11	k. 10	n. 8
c. 1	f. 2	i. 7	l. 7	o. 14

Multiple Choice

1. b	6. b	11. b	16. a	21. d	26. a
2. a	7. d	12. d	17. a	22. b	27. b
3. c	8. d	13. b	18. c	23. c	28. d
4. c	9. a	14. c	19. a	24. d	29. a
5. c	10. c	15. d	20. c	25. b	

Review of Concepts

1. true
2. high levels of negative emotion, a sense of uncontrollability, and self preoccupation
3. sudden
4. true
5. control
6. are out of the blue, and involve socially unacceptable and horrific themes
7. false
8. cleaning
9. false
10. anger or aggression
11. lumping; splitting
12. false
13. false
14. true
15. true
16. 50%
17. physiological hyperarousal; absence of positive affect
18. alcoholism
19. true

20. women
21. OCD
22. 95%
23. the elderly
24. false
25. loss; danger
26. anxiety sensitivity
27. parental indifference; physical abuse
28. insecure-anxious
29. extinguish; one; rare
30. false
31. are; are not
32. true
33. less
34. asleep
35. not sure
36. false
37. true
38. true
39. false
40. false
41. true
42. caffeine
43. true
44. prolonged exposure with response prevention
45. thinking; decatastrophizing
46. false
47. GAD; social phobia; specific phobia; OCD
48. true
49. true
50. false

Understanding Research

1. somatic; palpitations; tightness; light

2. carbon dioxide; control; panic

3. alone; mask; anxiety; lit; lap; no; 5; 15; 10; 20

4. panic attack; no illusion; illusion of control; twice; smothering; light; heart

5. interact; sufficient; control

6. No; social phobia; two treatments are not different; exposure treatment group will show more improvement than placebo or nondirective treatment

7. 5; 0 to 100; 85; 10

8. Because the average patient in the exposure group still has a score above the cut-off for identifying meaningful psychopathology.

CHAPTER 7
ACUTE AND POSTTRAUMATIC STRESS DISORDERS, DISSOCIATIVE DISORDERS, and SOMATOFORM DISORDERS

Chapter Outline

I. Overview

II. Acute and Posttraumatic Stress Disorders
- A. Typical Symptoms and Associated Features of ASD and PTSD
  - 1. Reexperiencing
  - 2. Avoidance
  - 3. Arousal or Anxiety
  - 4. Dissociative Symptoms
- B. Classification of Acute and Posttraumatic Stress Disorders
  - 1. Brief Historical Perspective
  - 2. Contemporary Classification
    - a. Acute Stress Disorder
    - b. Traumatic Events
    - c. Diagnostic Concerns
- C. Epidemiology of Trauma, Diagnostic Concerns, PTSD, and ASD
- D. Etiological Considerations and Research on PTSD and ASD
  - 1. Biological Factors in Traumatic Stress Disorders
    - a. Biological Effects of Exposure to Trauma
  - 2. Psychological Factors in Traumatic Stress Disorders
  - 3. Social Factors in Traumatic Stress Disorders
  - 4. Integration and Alternative Pathways
- E. Prevention and Treatment of ASD and PTSD
  - 1. Emergency Treatment of Trauma Survivors
  - 2. Treatment of PTSD
    - a. Therapeutic Reexposure to Trauma
  - 3. Long-Term Course and Outcome
    - a. Recovered Memories?

III. Dissociative Disorders
- A. Hysteria and Unconscious Mental Processes
  - 1. Charcot, Freud, and Janet
  - 2. Unconscious Mental Events in Contemporary Cognitive Science
  - 3. Hypnosis: Altered State or Social Role?
- B. Typical Symptoms of Dissociative Disorders
  - 1. Trauma and the Onset of Dissociative Symptoms
- C. Classification of Dissociative Disorders
  - 1. Brief Historical Perspective
  - 2. Contemporary Classification
  - 3. The Three Faces of Eve: The Case of Chris Sizemore

Learning Objectives

After reviewing the material presented in this chapter, you should be able to:

1. Define and list the DSM-IV symptoms of Posttraumatic Stress Disorder.

2. Distinguish PTSD from acute stress disorder and adjustment disorder.

3. Describe some of the treatment approaches utilized with patients with PTSD.

4. Distinguish dissociative and somatoform disorders.

5. Describe the views on hysteria of: early Greeks, Charcot, Janet, and Freud and compare these perspectives with the contemporary perspective.

6. Define dissociation and psychogenic amnesia.

7. Explain the connection between psychological trauma and fugue, amnesia, and multiple personality disorder.

8. Define retrograde, posttraumatic, anterograde, and selective amnesia.

9. Identify the DSM criteria for depersonalization disorder and dissociative identity disorder.

10. Define prosopagnosia and explain the significance of this biologically based disorder for the biological approach to dissociation.

11. Understand the psychological view of dissociative disorders, but be aware that little scientific research has been conducted to verify these theories.

12. Describe the ways in which hypnosis and abreaction presumably aid in the integration of dissociated memories.

13. Give the DSM-IV criteria for body dysmorphic disorder, hypochondriasis, somatization disorder, pain disorder, and conversion disorder.

14. Understand the way in which misdiagnosis of somatoform disorder can be dangerous.

15. Know Freud's theory of primary and secondary gain used to describe somatoform symptoms.

16. Describe the behavioural therapy approach to treatment of chronic pain.

17. Outline the way physicians should treat the patient who presents "excessive" physical concerns which are not physiologically based.

Key Terms — Matching #1

The following terms are important to know. To test your knowledge, match the following terms with their definitions. Answers are listed at the end of the chapter.

a. Traumatic stress
b. Acute Stress Disorder (ASD)
c. Posttraumatic stress disorder (PTSD)
d. Dissociative Disorders
e. Somatoform Disorders
f. Malingering
g. Factitious Disorder
h. Flashbacks
i. Depersonalization
j. Derealisation
k. Dissociative amnesia
l. Selective amnesia

m. Depersonalization disorder
n. Dissociative identity disorder
o. Multiple personality disorder
p. Hypnosis
q. Prosopagnosia
r. Retrospective reports
s. State-dependent learning
t. Iatrogenesis
u. Abreaction
v. Secondary victimization
w. Interpersonality amnesia
x. Priming

1. ____ a disorder characterized by the sudden inability to recall extensive and important personal information
2. ____ a sense of feeling cut off from oneself or one's environment
3. ____ impairment of face recognition sometimes resulting from brain damage
4. ____ characterized by persistent, maladaptive disruptions in the integration of memory, consciousness, or identity
5. ____ a marked sense of unreality about oneself or one's environment
6. ____ recollections about the past that have questionable reliability and validity
7. ____ an altered state of consciousness during which people are especially susceptible to suggestion
8. ____ occurs within 4 weeks of exposure to a trauma; characterized by dissociative symptoms, reexperiencing of the event, avoidance of reminders of the event, and anxiety or arousal
9. ____ lasts over a month after exposure to a trauma, or has a delayed onset (6 or more months after trauma); characterized by dissociative symptoms, reexperiencing of the event, avoidance of reminders of the event, and anxiety or arousal
10. ____ when professionals increase a rape survivor's emotional burden
11. ____ exposure to some event that involves actual or threatened death or serious injury to self or others
12. ____ the emotional reliving of a past traumatic experience
13. ____ a dissociative disorder characterized by the existence of two or more distinct personalities in a single individual, which repeatedly take over the person's behaviour outside of their awareness
14. ____ the previous term for dissociative identity disorder
15. ____ sudden, intrusive, vivid memories during which a trauma is replayed in images or thoughts
16. ____ pretending to have a psychological disorder in order to achieve some external gain
17. ____ pretending to have a psychological disorder in order to assume the sick role
18. ____ a dissociative disorder characterized by severe and persistent feelings of being detached from oneself
19. ____ learning that occurs in one state of affect or consciousness is recalled most accurately while in that same state
20. ____ a form of amnesia in which people do not lose their memory completely but are unable to remember only certain personal events and information
21. ____ characterized by unusual physical symptoms that occur in the absence of a known physical illness
22. ____ creation of a disorder by attempts at treatment
23. ____ showing a set of stimuli and later testing subjects with a degraded form of the stimuli
24. ____ lack of awareness of the experiences of one personality by an alter

Key Terms — Matching #2

The following terms are important to know. To test your knowledge, match the following terms with their definitions. Answers are listed at the end of the chapter.

1. Victimization
2. Two-factor theory
3. Trauma desensitization
4. Eye Movement Desensitization and Reprocessing (EMDR)
5. Recovered memories
6. False memories
7. Dissociative fugue
8. Hysteria
9. Amnesia
10. Psychogenic amnesia
11. Conversion disorder
12. Somatization disorder

13. La belle indifference
14. Briquet's syndrome
15. Hypochondriasis
16. Pain disorder
17. Body dysmorphic disorder
18. Diagnosis by exclusion
19. Primary gain
20. Secondary gain
21. Alexithymia
22. Thought suppression
23. Explicit memory
24. Implicit memory

a. _____ a pattern of response among survivors of violent crime that includes fear, guilt, self-blame, powerlessness, and lowered self-esteem

b. _____ a somatoform disorder characterized by preoccupying fear or belief that one is suffering from a physical illness, even in the face of a clean bill of health by a physician

c. _____ a somatoform disorder characterized by physical symptoms that mimic those found in neurological diseases, but which often do not make sense anatomically

d. _____ amnesia that is psychologically caused, resulting from trauma or emotional distress

e. _____ a process of identifying somatoform disorders by ruling out physical causes that could account for the symptoms

f. _____ avoidance of memories or thoughts of a trauma

g. _____ a controversial treatment using rapid back-and-forth eye movements to induce relaxation while reliving a traumatic event

h. _____ a somatoform disorder characterized by constant preoccupation with some imagined or grossly exaggerated defect in physical appearance

i. _____ dramatic recollections of a long-forgotten traumatic experience

j. _____ partial or complete loss of recall for a particular event or time period

k. _____ an unintentionally invented memory of an event that did not actually occur

l. _____ a psychoanalytic term that a symptom protects the ego from an unacceptable thought by serving as a symbolic, disguised expression of that thought

m. _____ a somatoform disorder characterized by multiple, somatic complaints in the absence of organic impairment

n. _____ a rare disorder characterized by sudden, unplanned travel, the inability to remember details about the past, and identity confusion or assumption of a new identity

o. _____ a psychoanalytic term that a symptom is rewarding because it allows a patient to avoid responsibility or elicit sympathy or attention from others

p. _____ a flippant lack of concern about the physical symptoms of a somatoform disorder

q. _____ an historic diagnostic category that included both dissociative and somatoform disorders; based on the ancient Greek idea that these symptoms were caused by a "dislodged, wandering uterus."

r. _____ a somatoform disorder characterized by preoccupation with pain in which psychological factors are involved

s. _____ explains the development of symptoms following trauma using a combination of classical and operant conditioning, whereby classical conditioning creates fears and operant conditioning maintains them

t. _____ treatment method where the client is first taught to relax, and while relaxed, gradually relives the traumatic event through discussion or fantasy

u   _____ a deficit in the capacity to recognize and express the emotions signaled by physiological arousal

v. _____ a name sometimes used to refer to somatization disorder

w. _____ changes in memory but with no conscious recollection

x. _____ conscious recollection of a past event

Names You Should Know — Matching

The following people have played an important role in research and theory of PTSD, dissociative, and somatoform disorders. To test your knowledge, match the following names with the descriptions of their contributions to the study of abnormal psychology. Answers are listed at the end of the chapter.

a. Pierre Janet
b. Harold Mersky
c. Nicholas Spanos
d. Jean Charcot
e. Sigmund Freud

1. _____ argued that multiple personalities are caused by role playing
2. _____ viewed dissociation as a normal process, similar to repression, whereby the ego defends itself against unacceptable thoughts
3. _____ used hypnosis to treat hysteria
4. _____ viewed dissociation as an abnormal process indicative of psychopathology
5. _____ argued that multiple personalities occur in response to leading questions asked by therapists.

Review of Concepts — Fill in the Blank and True/False

This section will help focus your studying by testing whether you understand the concepts presented in the text. After you have read and reviewed the material, test your comprehension and memory by filling in the following blanks or circling the right answer. Answers are listed at the end of the chapter.

1. PTSD is characterized by these three symptoms:_____, _____, and _____.

2. ASD is characterized by the above three symptoms and _____.

3. Sometimes the reexperiencing of PTSD and ASD occurs as a _____ state, which is usually brief.

4. In PTSD, avoidance may manifest as _____, where feelings seem dampened or nonexistent, and they withdraw from others.

5. Many people with PTSD and ASD are jumpy and nervous, showing an "exaggerated _____ response."

6. The development of ASD as a diagnostic category was in part an attempt to _____ the development of PTSD by providing early treatment.

7. What was wrong with earlier definitions of trauma? _____ _____.

8. What are five types of experience that often lead to the development of PTSD? _____, _____ _____, _____ and _____.

9. A woman cannot become pregnant as the result of a sexual assault:
   true   false

10. What three disorders commonly co-occur with PTSD? _____, _____, and _____.

11. It is thought that about _____% of women and _____% of men will develop PTSD at some point in their lives.

12. People who experience what type of trauma develop PTSD in the highest proportions? _____

13. People with a history of emotional problems are   **more   less**   likely to experience trauma and are   **more   less**   likely to develop PTSD.

14. There is evidence to suggest that some patients with PTSD dissociate, because they report low anxiety but tests show they have _____ arousal.

15. What are the three models that attempt to explain why not everybody that experiences a traumatic event develops PTSD? _____, _____, and _____.

16. Monozygotic (MZ) twins had a **higher** **lower** concordance rate than dizygotic (DZ) twins for experiencing trauma in the form of exposure to combat, and for developing PTSD symptoms in a study of Vietnam veterans.

17. Research suggests that high levels of thought _____ are associated with more severe symptoms of PTSD.

18. Research has suggested that an increase in the production of the neurotransmitter _____ in response to trauma causes the increased arousal and anxiety seen in PTSD, and that the increase in production of endogenous _____ in response to trauma causes the numbing.

19. One study showed that Vietnam veterans with PTSD showed **more** **less** pain sensitivity following exposure to a film of combat.

20. People cope **better** **worse** with trauma when they anticipate its onset.

21. What three characteristics of an attack increase the chance that survivors of sexual assault will develop PTSD? _____, _____, _____.

22. What three types of experiences among Vietnam veterans increase the risk of PTSD? _____, _____, and _____.

23. Social support **increases** **decreases** the risk for PTSD.

24. Research **supports** **does not support** the idea that immediate, emergency psychological treatment is effective in preventing PTSD.

25. According to a recent meta-analysis examining the effectiveness of various treatments for PTSD, _____ were found to be the most efficacious psychological therapies, and equally effective as _____,

the most effective drug therapies for PTSD. However, the psychological therapies were shown to have fewer_____ than the drug therapies.

26. Although painful and difficult, _____is the essential component of effective treatment for PTSD.

27. According to a recent meta-analysis on treatments for PTSD, EMDR was shown to be as efficacious as cognitive behavioural therapies: **true   false**

28. There is no evidence that repression of memories of traumatic events occurs:
    true   false

29. It is very difficult to establish whether a recovered memory is accurate:
    true   false

30. Freud viewed the unconscious mind as being   **dumb** or **smart**   while contemporary scientists view it as   **dumb** or   **smart**.

31. One study found that 80% of patients with dissociative identity disorder also met criteria for what disorder? _____.

32. What traumatic experience is hypothesized to play a role in the aetiology of many dissociative disorders? _____

33. Only 200 case histories of _____ disorder appeared in the entire world literature before 1980; a 1986 report suggested that about 6,000 cases of it had been diagnosed in North America alone, yet the diagnosis remains extremely rare in Europe and Japan.

34. Some professionals question the existence of dissociative identity disorder, arguing that it is created by the power of _____.

35. What is one important way that the multiple identity enactment created in laboratory studies differs from the multiple identities found in dissociative identity disorder?

_____

36. Patients with prosopagnosia demonstrate the normal preference for viewing faces that are familiar. This finding implies a dissociation between _____ and _____cognitive processes.

37. An adequate test of the hypothesized relation between child abuse and dissociative disorders requires _____ research following trauma survivors from childhood into adult life with assessments of dissociation at different times.

38. The evidence on genetic contribution to dissociative symptoms is currently _____.

39. Some psychologists argue that dissociative identity disorder is produced by iatrogenesis; in other words, who causes the disorder? _____

40. The goal of treatment for dissociative identity disorder is _____ _____.

41. What kind of professional do people with somatoform disorders typically see? _____.

42. Multisomatoform disorder has been proposed and requires _____ physical symptoms.

43. In one study, 27% of women undergoing what type of surgery actually suffered from somatization disorder? _____

44. Somatization disorder must have its onset in: **young adulthood**   **middle age**

45. Conversion disorders are   **more**   or   **less**   common now than in the past.

46. Somatization disorder is more common in which of the following: **women**   or **men**;   **blacks**   or   **whites**;   **less educated**   or   **more educated**

47. Somatoform disorders show high comorbidity with _____.

48. People with somatization disorder are more likely to have male relatives with _____disorder.

49. In one study, what percentage of patients diagnosed with conversion disorders were eventually found to have a neurological disease?   **5%**   **25%**   **45%**

50. Research has found that somatoform disorders are *NOT* more frequent in nonindustrialized countries: **true**   **false**

51. A recent study demonstrated that people with hypochondriasis and body dysmorphic disorder who are willing to _____ show improvement with cognitive-behavioural therapy.

Multiple Choice Questions

The following multiple choice questions will test your comprehension of the material presented in the chapter. Answers are listed at the end of the chapter.

1) Many people who suffer from PTSD also meet the diagnostic criteria for another mental disorder, particularly _____ and _____.

   a. depression; substance abuse
   b. hypomanic; antisocial personality disorder
   c. depression; adjustment disorder
   d. hypomanic; paranoid personality disorder

2) All of the following are cultural myths of sexual assault EXCEPT:

   a. women who are raped provoke it
   b. women who are raped seldom sustain physical injuries
   c. women who are raped often enjoy it
   d. many women who are raped are raped by an acquaintance

3) Jack, a Vietnam Veteran, runs for cover every time he hears an airplane pass by overhead. Jack's reaction can best be described as a:

   a. flashback   c. brief psychotic reaction
   b. dissociative state   d. hallucination

4) According to studies conducted in Canada and the U.S., women are more likely to develop PTSD, but men are _____ to report exposure to a traumatic event.

   a. more likely
   b. less likely
   c. just as likely
   d. under-report PTSD symptoms

5) According to one study conducted in Winnipeg, what percentage of people reporting exposure to trauma met the criteria for PTSD?

   a. 8%   c. 75%
   b. 25%   d. 88%

6) All of the following are factors that increase the risk for PTSD:

   a. having a history of emotional problems   c. being female
   b. being a minority group member   d. being wealthy

7) As many as _____ of all stranger rapes are not reported to authorities.

   a. one-third   c. one-quarter
   b. two-thirds   d. one-half

8) Some research indicates that it is helpful to recount stressful experiences because:

   a. it can reduce the various psychophysiological indicators of the stress response
   b. it helps dissipate negative feelings associated with the stressful experiences
   c. it helps the person "let go" of the experience and continue with his or her life
   d. there is no research that supports the effectiveness of recounting stressful experiences

9) A recent meta-analysis comparing psychological and pharmacological therapies for PTSD showed that:

   a. All psychological therapies were equally effective
   b. behavioural and cognitive behavioural therapies were the most effective.
   c. pharmacological treatments such as fluoxetine and sertraline were most effective.
   d. behavioural and cognitive behavioural therapies were just as effective as fluoxetine and sertraline, but the former therapies were associated with fewer treatment dropouts.

10) _____ is the help and understanding received from friends and family as well as from professionals.

   a. A personal network   c. Psychotherapy
   b. Social support   d. None of the above

11 Which of the following is NOT typically a symptom of PTSD?

   a. difficulty falling or staying asleep   c. paranoid thoughts or ideas
   b. irritability or outbursts of anger   d. difficulty concentrating

12) A horrifying experience that leads to general increases in anxiety and arousal, avoidance of emotionally charged situations, and the frequent reliving of the traumatic event is called:

   a. posttraumatic stress disorder   c. acute stress disorder
   b. victimization   d. generalized anxiety disorder

13) Sudden, unplanned travel, the inability to remember certain past details, and confusion about one's identity are primary features of:

   a. general amnesia
   b. Briquet's syndrome

   c. body dysmorphic disorder
   d. dissociative fugue

14) Abnormal fears of having a serious medical disorder, even after a thorough medical evaluation reveals nothing wrong, is characteristic of:

   a. hypochondriasis
   b. depersonalization disorder

   c. somatization disorder
   d. conversion disorder

15) This term is used to describe people who habitually and deliberately pretend to have a physical illness.

   a. hypochondriasis
   b. psychosis

   c. factitious disorder
   d. adjustment disorder

16) An unfortunate consequence of having a somatoform disorder is:

   a. the patient does not attend to the medical aspects of the disorder, resulting in underutilization of health care
   b. the psychological nature of the patient's problems go unnoticed, and unnecessary medical procedures are performed
   c. the seriousness of the physical complaints are overlooked, and necessary medical treatments are refused
   d. mental health professionals are consulted instead of physicians, resulting in poor physical health care

17) Which disorder does NOT appear to overlap with somatoform disorders?

   a. anxiety disorders
   b. depression

   c. antisocial personality disorder
   d. multiple personality disorder

18) Freud believed that both dissociative and somatoform disorders were:

   a. expressions of unresolved anger
   b. reactions of the superego toward repressed impulses
   c. expressions of unconscious conflict
   d. conscious reactions to traumatic situations

19) "La belle indifference" is occasionally exhibited by patients with:

   a. multiple personality disorder
   b. pain disorder

   c. psychogenic amnesia
   d. somatization disorder

20) Whenever Tom looks into the mirror, the first thing he notices is his large and some-what pointed ears. Although friends have reassured him otherwise, he is convinced that his ears are the first thing others notice about him, too. In fact, he wonders whether some people may call him Mr. Spock behind his back. He has consulted with several plastic surgeons and his first surgery has just been scheduled. Tom displays symptoms of:

a. somatization disorder
b. Briquet's syndrome
c. conversion disorder
d. body dysmorphic disorder

21) Sally is depressed about her relationship with her boyfriend as she studies for her spring chemistry final. The next fall, she takes another chemistry course and easily remembers the material from her spring course while studying for her first quiz. She is also depressed now due to a fight with her girlfriend. This is:

a. state-dependent learning
b. abreaction
c. hypnotic recall
d. recovered memory

22) How might antianxiety, antipsychotic, or antidepressant medications be helpful in the treatment of dissociative disorders?

a. they facilitate reintegration of the dissociated states
b. they reduce the level of the patient's emotional distress
c. they increase the likelihood of having one personality become dominant over other personalities
d. they are not recommended treatment for dissociative disorders

23) A critical consideration in the diagnosis of a somatoform disorder is that the person:

a. may be aware of the psychological factors producing the disorder
b. may minimize their physical complaints, resulting in not detecting the disorder
c. may also have coexisting multiple personalities
d. may actually have a real but as yet undetected physical illness

24) Which disorder is NOT a type of somatoform disorder?

a. depersonalization disorder
b. body dysmorphic disorder
c. conversion disorder
d. pain disorder

25) A distinguishing feature of somatization disorder is:

a. the physical complaints involve multiple somatic systems (e.g., gastrointestinal, cardiovascular, reproductive)
b. the physical complaints are limited to only one somatic system
c. the patient appears very serious, obsessive, and emotionally withdrawn
d. the onset of the disorder rarely occurs before age 30

26) The separation of mental processes such as memory or consciousness that are usually integrated is referred to as:

   a. abreaction
   b. dissociation
   c. repression
   d. deja vu

27) Which of the following is the best definition of a conversion symptom?

   a. a physical symptom in one part of the body that is actually referred pain or trauma from another part of the body
   b. a symptom produced by psychological conflict that mimics a symptom found in a neurological disease
   c. a symptom produced by injury which is exacerbated by psychological conflict
   d. an emotional symptom such as depressed mood produced by physical trauma

28) When is the diagnosis of a dissociative disorder NOT appropriate?

   a. when the patient has a history of child sexual abuse
   b. when the dissociative process is abrupt in onset
   c. when the patient additionally reports feeling depressed
   d. when the dissociation occurs in the presence of substance abuse or organic pathology

29) Joe, a housepainter, reports to his family doctor that he has not been able to work for six months because of pain in his legs. In fact, he can barely walk to the kitchen from his bedroom because of the pain. No injury occurred that would explain the situation. His wife has been taking care of him but is very concerned about the financial strain this is causing. His doctor orders a thorough examination. If nothing is found, what diagnosis should his doctor consider?

   a. conversion disorder
   b. hypochondriasis
   c. pain disorder
   d. somatoform disorder

30) The onset of a dissociative episode:

   a. is typically abrupt and precipitated by a traumatic event
   b. is slow and insidious in nature
   c. can be traced to certain metabolic deficiencies
   d. typically happens following a severe head injury

31) A conversion symptom that serves the function of protecting the conscious mind by expressing the conflict unconsciously is referred to as:

   a. la belle indifference
   b. primary gain
   c. diagnosis by exclusion
   d. abreaction

32) While both disorders involve memory loss, a major difference between dissociative amnesia and dissociative fugue is that:

    a. dissociative fugue is characterized by sudden and unexpected travel away from home
    b. the memory loss in dissociative amnesia has a physical basis
    c. dissociative amnesia is characterized by the emergence of at least one additional personality
    d. dissociative fugue additionally includes persistent feelings of being detached from oneself

33) Research on the prevalence of somatoform disorders suggests that they:

    a. appear to be more common than depression in the general population
    b. appear to be less common during war time
    c. appear to be rare in the general population
    d. have increased in prevalence since Freud's time

34) The sociocultural view of the aetiology of somatoform disorders suggests that:

    a. people with education and financial security have greater access to physicians who will listen to their somatic complaints
    b. people in nonindustrialised societies have a greater sense of community and are more likely to describe their inner distress to others in their social network
    c. people in industrialized societies have more opportunity to develop a more sophisticated vocabulary for their physical symptoms
    d. people with less education or financial security have less opportunity to learn how to describe their inner turmoil in psychological terms

35) A person with which of the following would be at risk for developing a dissociative disorder?

    a. a family history of depression   c. a history of violent behaviour
    b. a history of child sexual abuse   d. all of the above

36) Why are people with somatoform disorders likely to reject a referral to a mental health professional from their physicians?

    a. people may have difficulty accepting the possibility of the psychological basis to their physical symptoms
    b. people may feel that their physician is belittling their problems
    c. people may feel that their physician is not being empathic
    d. all of the above

37) Which statement is NOT correct about somatization disorder?

    a. it is more common among higher socioeconomic groups
    b. it is more common among women
    c. it is more common among African Americans than whites
    d. somatic symptoms are more frequent among people who have lost a spouse

38) Every Friday, Sarah's fifth grade class has a spelling test. Every Friday morning, she complains of a stomachache to her mother. This may be an example of:

    a. expressing an emotional concern that has a genuine emotional basis
    b. expressing an emotional concern in terms of a physical complaint
    c. expressing a physical complaint that has been reinforced by the environment
    d. expressing a psychological symptom that has an organic basis

39) Somatoform disorders are characterized by:

    a. physical complaints that can be traced to organic impairment
    b. patients who deliberately lie about the presence of physical symptoms
    c. physical symptoms that cannot be explained on the basis of underlying physical illness
    d. physical symptoms which are consciously linked to psychological difficulties

40) Although their presenting symptoms differ greatly in appearance, a common link between dissociative and somatoform disorders is:

    a. both involve memory loss
    b. both require extensive medical treatment
    c. both apparently involve unconscious processes
    d. all of the above

41) In contrast to Freud, contemporary cognitive scientists:

    a. do not recognize the existence of unconscious processes
    b. believe that unconscious processes are much less influential in shaping both normal and abnormal behaviour
    c. believe that unconscious processes are more influential than conscious processes in shaping both normal and abnormal behaviour
    d. have a much less restricted view of unconscious processes and their role in shaping behaviour

42) The analogue experiments conducted by Spanos and his colleagues on the symptoms of dissociative identity disorder suggest that:

    a. hypnosis had no relationship to the presence of symptoms of this disorder
    b. they disappeared under hypnosis
    c. they can be induced through role-playing and hypnosis
    d. experimental hypnosis increases risk for dissociative identity disorder

43) An example of a sociological theory of the cause of dissociative identity disorder is

    a. it is caused by disturbances in the temporal lobe of the brain
    b. it is caused by a perceptual disturbance that impairs the ability to recognize faces
    c. it is produced by iatrogenesis, specifically, through the leading questions of therapists
    d. it is produced by recovered memories of the loss of a parent

44) Which of the following is not a characteristic of hypnosis?

    a. people vary in how easy they are to hypnotize
    b. some researchers feel that it is simply a social role
    c. it is usually intentionally faked
    d. hypnosis can have powerful effects

Understanding Research — Fill in the Blank

Implicit Memory in Dissociative Identity Disorder: The text presents a detailed description of a study by Eric Eich et al in the Research Close-Up. Finding the answers to these questions will help you get a good understanding of this study and why it is important. It is not necessary to memorize the answers; the process of finding them in the textbook will help you learn the material you need to know.

1. There is debate about whether dissociative identity disorder is _____ or real. Implicit memory tasks assess subtle mental processes that are _____ to feign.

2. The study used two tasks: reading and rating a set of words and reviewing a series of partial but increasingly complete _____ until they were identified. Participants later were presented with word _____ corresponding with the earlier words and repeated the partial _____.

3. One _____ was primed and the _____ was tested for _____ memory effects.

4. Priming effects in the word test were stronger when they were conducted within the same _____. However, there were no differences on the _____ completion task. _____ between personalities does occur but is not _____.

5. Scientists are skeptical about the accuracy of people's memories of the past, even when people report them _____ and _____. Research designs using _____ reports are preferred over those using _____ reports.

6. One problem is normal limitations of _____. The second is that memories of people with _____ problems are particularly unreliable. The third is that psychopathology systematically _____ people's memories. Memory processes are said to be "mood-_____." This could lead researchers to speculate that depressed people who remember more _____ experiences are depressed because they had more sad experiences, when really they may have had the same number of sad experiences but just _____ more when asked to report on them.

7. One study suggests that memory for _____ events is fairly reliable, but that people _____ their history with regard to more global experiences. _____ report more negative memories of the past than do _____. Research evidence does not support the hypothesis that memories are _____ congruent, specifically among depressed people.

8. Freud was uncertain whether to believe his patients' memories of _____ _____. In the end he decided they were _____. Current research indicates that Freud was probably _____. The conclusion of the section is that: _____ _____.

Brief Essay

As a final exercise, write out answers to the following brief essay questions. Then compare your answers with the material presented in the text.

After you have answered these questions, review the "critical thinking" questions that are presented at the end of the text chapter. Answering these questions will help you integrate important issues and themes that have been featured throughout the chapter.

1. Briefly describe Posttraumatic Stress Disorder (PTSD). Give an example of an experience that may result in PTSD and identify the various symptoms that might accompany this disorder.

2. While some professionals believe that multiple personalities are real and more com-
    mon than previously thought, others believe that the condition is no more than role-
    playing. Discuss this controversy, citing the research and clinical evidence that
    supports both points of view.

3. Are recovered memories examples of dissociation or are they produced through
    the power of suggestion? Defend your own position on this controversial topic.

4. Review the methodological concerns surrounding the use of retrospective reports.
    What are the important questions that have been raised regarding their reliability
    and validity? What are the implications of these concerns regarding the use of ret-
    rospective reports in research?

5. If you are a primary care physician with a patient who has a number of vague and
    inconsistent physical complaints, but an extensive medical evaluation reveals no
    organic pathology, what types of questions would you consider in trying to deter-
    mine whether the patient has a somatoform disorder? How would you approach
    the treatment of this patient if a diagnosis of somatization disorder was given?

ANSWER KEY

Key Terms — Matching #1

1. k	7. p	13. n	19. s
2. i	8. b	14. o	20. l
3. q	9. c	15. h	21. e
4. d	10. v	16. f	22. t
5. j	11. a	17. g	23. x
6. r	12. u	18. m	24. w

Names You Should Know

1. c
2. e
3. d
4. a
5. b

Key Terms — Matching #2

a. 1	g. 4	m. 12	s. 2
b. 15	h. 17	n. 7	t. 3
c. 11	i. 5	o. 20	u. 21
d. 10	j. 9	p. 13	v. 14
e. 18	k. 6	q. 8	w. 24
f. 22	l. 19	r. 16	x. 25

Multiple Choice

1. a	4. a	7. b	10. b	13. d
2. d	5. a	8. a	11. c	14. a
3. b	6. d	9. d	12. a	15. c

16.	b	22.	b	28.	d	34.	d	40.	c
17.	d	23.	d	29.	c	35.	b	41.	b
18.	c	24.	a	30.	a	36.	d	42.	c
19.	d	25.	a	31.	b	37.	a	43.	c
20.	d	26.	b	32.	a	38.	b	44.	c
21.	a	27.	b	33.	c	39.	c		

Review of Concepts

1. reexperiencing, avoidance, and arousal or anxiety
2. dissociative symptoms
3. dissociative
4. numbing of responsiveness
5. startle
6. prevent
7. they defined trauma as outside usual experience but trauma is not that rare
8. war, rape, child sexual abuse, spouse abuse, witnessing disasters
9. false
10. depression, anxiety disorders, substance abuse
11. 10%; 5%
12. rape
13. more;   more
14. high
15. threshold; diathesis-stress; illness
16. higher
17. suppression
18. norepinephrine; opioids
19. less
20. better
21. rape is completed; if they were physically injured; if their life was threatened
22. being wounded; being involved in death of civilians; witnessing atrocities
23. decreases
24. supports

25. behavioural and cognitive-behavioural; fluoxetine and sertraline; treatment dropouts
26. reexposure
27. true
28. false
29. true
30. smart; dumb
31. PTSD
32. child sexual abuse
33. dissociative identity
34. suggestion
35. amnesia is absent in the enactment but typical in the disorder
36. conscious and unconscious
37. prospective
38. inconclusive
39. a therapist
40. to reintegrate the personalities into one
41. physician
42. fewer
43. hysterectomy
44. young adulthood
45. less
46. women; blacks; less educated
47. depression
48. antisocial personality
49. 25%
50. true
51. accept a referral for psychological counselling

Understanding Research

1. fake; difficult

2. drawings; stems; drawings

3. personality; alter; implicit

4. personality; picture; amnesia; complete

5. readily; confidently; prospective; retrospective

6. memory; emotional; biases; congruent; sad; remember

7. specific; rewrite; children; parents; mood

8. sexual abuse; fantasies; wrong; Retrospective reports of specific past events are reliable and valid enough to use a first, less expensive research method.

CHAPTER 8
STRESS AND PHYSICAL HEALTH

Chapter Outline

I. Overview

II. Stress
    A. Defining Stress
        1. Stress as a Stimulus
        2. Stress as a Response
        3. Stress as a Stimulus-Response Combination
    B. Typical Symptoms and Associated Features
        1. Physiological Responses to Stress
            a. Damage due to Chronic Stress
            b. Immune Function
            c. Physiological Toughness?
        2. Emotional Responses to Stress
        3. Cognitive Responses to Stress
        4. Behavioral Responses to Stress
        5. Health Behavior
    C. Classification of Stress and Physical Illness
        1. Brief Historical Perspective
        2. Contemporary Approaches
        3. Illness as a Cause of Stress
        4. Canadian Focus: Endler's Multidimensional Interaction Model of Stress, Anxiety, and Coping

III. The Role of Psychological Factors in Some Familiar Illnesses
    A. Cancer
    B. Acquired Immune Deficiency Syndrome (AIDS)
    C. Pain Management
    D. Sleep Disorders

IV. Cardiovascular Disease
    A. Typical Symptoms and Associated Features of Hypertension and CHD
    B. Classification of CVD
    C. Epidemiology of CVD
        1. Risk Factors for CHD
        2. Risk Factors for Hypertension
    D. Aetiological Considerations and Research on CVD
        1. Biological Factors in CVD
        2. Psychological Factors in CVD
            a. Cardiovascular Reactivity to Stress

b. Life Stressors and CVD: Job Strain
c. Type A Behavior and Hostility
d. Depression and Anxiety
3. Social Factors in CVD
4. Integration and Alternative Pathways
E. Prevention and Treatment of Cardiovascular Disease
1. Primary Prevention
2. Secondary Prevention
3. Tertiary Prevention

Learning Objectives

After reviewing the material presented in this chapter, you should be able to:

1. Define stress, stress as a stimulus, stress as a response, and stress as a stimulus-response combination.

2. Know what is meant by general adaptation syndrome.

3. Distinguish between Cannon's and Selye's theories regarding the way in which stress causes illness.

4. Define physiological toughness.

5. Compare problem-focused and emotion-focused coping with stress.

6. Describe the emotional, cognitive, and behavioral responses to stress.

7. Understand how stress is used in classification in DSM-IV.

8. Understand the role of psychological factors in cancer, AIDS, and in problems with pain.

9. Distinguish primary and secondary hypertension.

10. Describe the major causes of primary hypertension.

11. Understand the impact of low control, high demand job strain on hypertension.

12. Understand therelationship between depression and anxiety, and CHD.

13. Describe the major characteristics of the Type A personality and the current thinking about its role in coronary heart disease.

14. Understand the primary preventive, secondary preventive and tertiary preventive treatment approaches which are successful in treatment and prevention of cardio-vascular disease.

Key Terms - Matching #1

The following terms related to stress and physical health are important to know. To test your knowledge, match the following terms with their definitions. Answers are listed at the end of the chapter.

a. Stress
b. Traumatic stress
c. Psychosomatic disorders
d. Behavioral medicine
e. Health psychologists
f. General adaptation syndrome
g. Primary appraisal
h. Secondary appraisal
i. Optimism
j. Fight or flight response

k. Sleep terror disorder
l. Sleepwalking disorder
m. Specificity hypothesis
n. Carcinogens
o. Cardiovascular disease (CVD)
p. Hypertension
q. Coronary heart disease (CHD)
r. Myocardial infarction (MI)
s. Systolic blood pressure

1. ____ an individual's cognitive evaluation of the challenge, threat, or harm posed by a particular event
2. ____ a challenging event that requires physiological, cognitive, or behavioral adaptation
3. ____ a disorder involving abrupt awakening and intense autonomic arousal but little memory of a dream and a quick return to sleep
4. ____ a group of diseases of the heart
5. ____ an individual's assessment of his or her abilities and resources for coping with a difficult event
6. ____ a general cognitive style of taking a positive attitude
7. ____ a three-stage model of reaction to stress involving alarm, resistance, and exhaustion
8. ____ a heart attack, the most deadly form of CHD, caused by oxygen deprivation and death of heart muscle tissue
9. ____ stress caused by exposure to catastrophic event involving actual or threatened death to oneself or others
10. ____ high blood pressure
11. ____ a multidisciplinary field including medical and mental health professionals who investigate psychological factors in the symptoms, etiology, and treatment of physical illness
12. ____ specific personality types cause specific psychosomatic diseases
13. ____ the highest blood pressure reading, it is the pressure that the blood exerts against the arteries when the heart is beating
14. ____ a response to threat in which psychophysiological reactions prepare the body to take action against danger
15. ____ a disorder involving rising during sleep and walking about in an unresponsive state with no later memory of the episode
16. ____ a term indicating that physical disease is a product of both the mind and body

17. _____ a group of disorders affecting the heart and circulatory system
18. _____ cancer-causing agents
19. _____ psychologists who specialize in behavioral medicine

Key Terms — Matching #2

The following terms related to stress and physical health are important to know. To test your knowledge, match the following terms with their definitions. Answers are listed at the end of the chapter.

1. Psychoneuroimmunology
2. Glucocorticoids
3. T cells
4. Lymphocytes
5. Antigens
6. Immunosuppression
7. Physiological toughness
8. Problem-focused coping
9. Emotion-focused coping
10. Diastolic blood pressure
11. Angina pectoris

12. Sudden cardiac death (SCD)
13. Secondary hypertension
14. Essential hypertension
15. Myocardial ischemia
16. Atherosclerosis
17. Coronary occlusion
18. Cardiovascular reactivity
19. Type A behavior pattern
20. Acquired immune deficiency syndrome (AIDS)
21. Human immunodeficiency virus (HIV)

a. _____ hypertension resulting from a known problem such as a diagnosed kidney or endocrine disorder
b. _____ the decreased production of immune agents, often a result of stress
c. _____ a competitive, hostile, urgent, impatient, achievement-striving style of responding to challenge
d. _____ sudden oxygen deprivation when arteries are completely blocked by fatty deposits or when blood clots make their way to the heart muscle
e. _____ internally oriented coping involving attempts to alter subjective distress
f. _____ a category of white blood cells that fight off antigens
g. _____ a form of high blood pressure where the hypertension is the principal disorder
h. _____ externally oriented coping that involves attempts to change a stressor
i. _____ temporary oxygen deprivation that accompanies intermittent chest pains which causes no permanent damage
j. _____ a beneficial effect of stress under certain circumstances
k. _____ death within 24 hours of a coronary episode
l. _____ a measure of the intensity of an individual's cardiovascular reactions to stress in the laboratory which predicts future cardiovascular disease
m. _____ a major form of coronary heart disease involving intermittent chest pains brought on by some form of exertion
n. _____ adrenal hormones secreted in response to stress
o. _____ foreign substances like bacteria that invade the body

p. _____ the lowest blood pressure reading, it is the pressure that the blood exerts against the arteries between heartbeats

q. _____ research on the effects of stress on the functioning of the immune system

r. _____ one of the major types of white blood cells of the immune system

s. _____ the thickening of the coronary artery wall as a result of the accumulation of blood lipids with age

t. _____ the virus that causes AIDS

u. _____ an infectious disease which attacks the immune system

Key Terms — Matching #3

The following terms are related to stress and physical health and are important to know. To test your knowledge, match the following terms with their definitions. Answers are listed at the end of the chapter.

a. Health behavior
b. Primary sleep disorder
c. Dyssomnias
d. Parasomnias
e. Primary insomnia
f. Narcolepsy
g. Breathing-related sleep disorder
h. Circadian rhythm sleep disorder
i. Nightmare disorder
j. Longitudinal study

k. Cross-sectional approach
l. Social ecology
m. Antihypertensives
n. Beta blockers
o. Stress management
p. Biofeedback
q. Role playing
r. Primary hypersomnia
s. Sleep apnea

1. _____ activities essential to promoting good health, such as healthy eating, exercise, and avoidance of unhealthy activities like drug use

2. _____ a disorder involving frequent awakening to alertness by terrifying dreams

3. _____ disorders characterized by abnormal events that occur during sleep, like nightmares

4. _____ the interrelations between the individual and the social world

5. _____ the disruption of sleep due to breathing problems such as sleep apnea, the temporary obstruction of the respiratory airway

6. _____ a treatment to teach more effective coping skills, reduce adverse reactions to stress and improve health behavior

7. _____ medications effective in reducing high blood pressure

8. _____ a type of research design in which subjects are studied over time, allowing researchers to make inferences about causation

9. _____ drugs that reduce the risk of myocardial infarction of sudden coronary death

10. _____ irresistible attacks of refreshing sleep

11. _____ a mismatch between the patient's 24-hour sleeping patterns and their 24-hour life demands

12. _____ a condition where sleeping disturbance is the primary complaint

13. ____ a technique used in therapy of improvisational play acting to teach patients how to respond to stressful interactions with less hostility
14. ____ problems in the amount, quality, or timing of sleep
15. ____ a treatment using equipment to monitor physiological processes and provide the patient with feedback about them to help patients gain conscious control over them
16. ____ research design in which subjects are studied at one point in time
17. ____ excessive sleepiness characterized by prolonged or daytime sleep which interferes with functioning
18. ____ difficulties initiating or maintaining sleep, or poor quality of sleeping
19. ____ a sleep disorder caused by temporary obstruction of the airway

Names You Should Know — Matching

The following people have played an important role in research and theory on stress and health. To test your knowledge, match the following names with the descriptions of their contributions to the study of abnormal psychology. Answers are listed at the end of the chapter.

      a. Richard Lazarus   b. Hans Selye   c. Walter Cannon

1. ____ a McGill University psychologist who defined stress in terms of the general adaptation syndrome; did much research on animal analogue studies of the GAS
2. ____ argued that stress is not just a stimulus but also the individual's response to the stimulus, specifically their cognitive appraisal of the event as being potentially harmful and exceeding their coping resources
3. ____ one of the first researchers to conduct systematic studies of stress; interested in the fight or flight response

Review of Concepts — Fill in the Blank and True/False

This section will help focus your studying by testing whether you understand the concepts presented in the text. After you have read and reviewed the material, test your comprehension and memory by filling in the following blanks or circling the right answer. Answers are listed at the end of the chapter.

1. Stress can be produced by daily _____ as well as by traumatic events.

2. Scientists used to think that psychological factors were   **important** or **irrelevant** in most physical illnesses; today they think they are   **important** or **irrelevant**.

3. The Diagnostic and Statistical Manual no longer contains a list of psychosomatic disorders because_____.

4. Holmes and Rahe developed the Social Readjustment Rating Scale, an attempt to measure the amount of _____ caused by various life events.

5. List three criticisms of the Social Readjustment Rating Scale:

   _____

   _____

   _____

6. What are the three stages of the GAS? _____,

   _____, and _____

7. One problem with Lazarus' approach to defining stress is that it runs the risk of being tautological, or _____.

8. The fight or flight response is _____ in the modern world.

9. Research indicates that optimism **is**   **is not**   linked to better health habits and less illness.

10. An analogy for **Cannon's** or **Selye's** theory is a car in which the engine continues to race instead of idling down after running fast, and an analogy for **Cannon's** or **Selye's** theory is a car that has run out of gas and is damaged because stress keeps turning the key, trying to restart the engine.

11. Another mechanism whereby stress may cause physical illness is the stress response sapping _____ away from routine bodily functions.

12. Stress weakens immune functioning: **true**   **false**

13. In one study with newly married couples, partners who were more _____ during discussions of marital problems showed greater immunosuppression during the next 24 hours.

14. Heightened immune functioning is **adaptive** or **maladaptive** in response to immediate threat from an evolutionary perspective.

15. One theory indicates that the moderate release of **betablockers** or **epinephrine and norepinephrine** serves to protect the body from depletion under future, more intense stress, a process called physiological toughness.

16. People who repress their anxiety show fewer psychophysiological reactions to stress: **true**   **false**

17. Predictability of a stressor   **improves**   or   **impairs**   our ability to cope with it.

18. Rats who can stop a shock by pressing a bar experience a bigger stress response than rats who receive an identical shock but don't have to worry about stopping it: **true**   **false**

19. One pathway that may explain how stress and illness are linked is that stress can reduce people's _____.

20. The more a stressed monkey can interact with other monkeys, the less immuno-suppression it demonstrates: **true**   **false**

21. Stress can cause illness, but illness can also cause _____.

22. Modern research supports the specificity hypothesis, that certain personality types are more prone to certain psychosomatic illnesses: **true**   **false**

23. Why does the DSM-IV not include the rating system for severity of stressors that-was included in DSM-III and DSM-III-R? _____.

24. Cancer deaths have substantially decreased over the past 20 years: **true**   **false**

25. Cancer is the leading cause of death today: **true**   **false**

26. Stress can directly affect the body's ability to fight cancer cells: **true**   **false**

27. Psychological treatments, such as structured self-help groups, have unfortunately not been shown to be effective in reducing the death rate among cancer patients: **true**   **false**

28. The prevalence of HIV/AIDS is particularly high on which continent? _____.

29. Although annual rates of HIV cases are slowly decreasing in Canada, rates are rising in   **men**   or   **women**.

30. Rates of HIV cases are also rapidly rising amongst which ethnic group in Canada? _____

31. Programs to educate the public about how HIV is transmitted are quite effective in changing risky behaviors related to transmission: **true**   **false**

32. A wide range of treatments, such as biofeedback, hypnosis, relaxation training, and cognitive therapy are quite useful in eliminating chronic pain: **true**   **false**

33. Cardiovascular disease is the third leading cause of death in the United States: **true**   **false**

34. Why is hypertension called the "silent killer"? _____

35. The rate of death due to CVD has decreased in the United States in recent years: **true**   **false**

36. Where has the rate of death due to CVD increased? _____

37. Who are more likely to suffer from CHD?   **men**   **women**

38. Who are more likely to suffer from CHD: people from   **low**   or   **high**   income groups?

39. Which of the following are not among the risk factors for CHD?
    drinking   **smoking**   **obesity**   **a fatty diet**

40. The nature of the relationship between age and risk for CHD is identical for men and women: **true**   **false**

41. Rats with a genetic predisposition to develop hypertension do so only when exposed to salty diets or environmental stress: **true**   **false**

42. The Los Angeles earthquake was linked to **higher**   or **lower** levels of cardiac deaths.

43. Job strain involves a situation with **high**   or **low** psychological demand with **high**   or   **low**   decisional control.

44. The number of _____ a woman has increases her risk for heart disease if she works but not if she is a homemaker.

45. The key feature of the Type A behavior pattern in predicting CHD is
    _____.

46. Depression **is** or **is not** correlated with CHD.

47. The only two treatment conditions that lowered blood pressure in a study comparing 1) weight reduction, 2) salt reduction, 3) stress management, 4) calcium supplement, 5) magnesium supplement, 6) potassium supplement, and 7) fish oil supplement, were: _____.

48. A recent meta-analysis comparing various psychosocial interventions in cardiac rehabilitation concluded that interventions such as _____ for anxiety or anger reduction, or _____, are useful in reducing emotional distress, blood pressure, heart rate, and cholesterol levels, and are associated with a lower incidence of _____.

Multiple Choice Questions

The following multiple choice questions will test your comprehension of the material presented in the chapter. Answers are listed at the end of the chapter.

1) All of the following are criticisms of the Holmes and Rahe Social Re-Adjustment Rating Scale EXCEPT:

 a. the inclusion of both positive and negative events as stressors
 b. failure to distinguish between transient and chronic life events
 c. a given stressor does not always produce the same number of life change units for all individuals in all situations
 d. all of the above are criticisms of this scale

2) Generally, hypertension is defined by a systolic blood pressure of above _____ and a diastolic blood pressure of above _____.

 a. 110; 60
 b. 120; 70
 c. 130; 80
 d. 140; 90

3) According to Walter Cannon, _____ is the mobilization of the body in reaction to a perceived threat.

 a. stage of alarm
 b. generalized arousal
 c. emergency response
 d. physiological toughness

4) Which of the following is NOT a reaction of the body to sympathetic nervous system arousal?

 a. heart rate increases
 b. blood pressure rises
 c. blood sugar lowers
 d. respiration rate increases

5) Although somewhat stressful, _____ decreases negative responding to an actual stressor.

a. predictability
b. anticipation
c. control
d. appraisal

6) Anxiety, depression, and _____ are considered to be the primary affective responses to stressors.

a. anger
b. tension
c. an upset stomach
d. aggression

7) Stress plays a role in:

a. all physical disorders
b. some physical disorders
c. only heart disease
d. no physical disorders

8) _____ of all deaths from CHD occur within 24 hours of a coronary event.

a. One-quarter
b. One-half
c. One-third
d. Two-thirds

9) Which would have the greatest risk for suffering from high blood pressure?
a. a male who is homeless
b. a male who is a stock broker
c. a female who is an attorney
d. a female who is a homemaker

10) This uses laboratory equipment to monitor physiological processes that generally occur outside of conscious awareness to help individuals learn how to control their autonomic nervous system functions voluntarily.

a. biofeedback
b. stress management
c. systematic desensitization
d. flooding

11) _____ is the most important goal of intervention with cardiovascular disease.

a. Medication
b. Prevention
c. Psychotherapy
d. Education

12) According to the Social Re-Adjustment Rating Scale, _____ is the most significant life event that constitutes the greatest number of life change units.

a. pregnancy
b. divorce
c. foreclosure of a mortgage or loan
d. death of one's spouse

13) Psychoneuroimmunology refers to the study of:

    a. decreased production of T cells and other immune agents
    b. inhibition and destruction of various immune agents
    c. the effects of stress on the functioning of the immune system
    d. white blood cells that fight off foreign substances that invade the body

14) Psychologists in this field define disease as "dis-ease", indicating that illness is a departure not only from adaptive biological functioning but also from adaptive social and psychological functioning.

    a. biopsychosocial psychology   c. health psychology
    b. behavioral psychology   d. dynamic psychology

15) Which is not a method of transmitting HIV:

    a. donating blood   c. sexual intercourse
    b. needle-sharing   d. mother to fetus

16) According to the Framingham Study, which was reviewed in your textbook, which of the following is most likely to suffer from heart disease?

    a. a woman who is a homemaker and has two children
    b. a woman who is a homemaker and has four children
    c. a woman who is a sales manager and has two children
    d. a woman who is a waitress and has four children

17) This term indicates that physical disease is a product of both the mind and body.

    a. somatoform   c. dissociative
    b. cognitive error   d. psychosomatic

18) All of the following are examples of cognitive responses to stress EXCEPT:

    a. control   c. appraisal
    b. repression   d. predictability

Understanding Research — Fill in the Blank

Canadian Focus: Endler's Multidimensional Interaction Model of Stress, Anxiety, and Coping: Endler's work builds on ideas developed by Richard Lazarus; however, Endler's model emphasizes the importance of interactions among key variables. Finding the answers to these questions will help you get a good understanding of this study and why it is important. It is not necessary to memorize the answers; the process of finding them in the textbook will help you learn the material you need to know.

1. Trait anxiety is a key variable that is central to Endler's model. Trait anxiety is defined as one's proneness or predisposition to experience _____. Endler proposes that there are four types of trait anxiety which are defined by the sorts of stressors that produce anxiety: _____, _____, _____, and _____. Of the studies that have tested Endler's interactional model, _____ supported the model. One study assessed state and trait anxiety in military personnel in threatening and non-threatening situations. The dependent measure in this study was _____. There were two independent measures in the study, a grouping variable _____ and an experimental condition _____. Support for the model was derived by showing that state anxiety was determined by an interaction between these two independent variables.

2. Endler also proposes that coping styles and stressors interact to increase state anxiety. Three sorts of coping are: _____, _____, and _____. This aspect of his model has particularly important implications for understanding how people cope with _____.

Disclosure of Trauma and Immunity: The text presents a detailed description of a study by Pennebaker, Kiecolt-Glaser, and Glaser in the Research Close-Up. Finding the answers to these questions will help you get a good understanding of this study and why it is important. It is not necessary to memorize the answers; the process of finding them in the textbook will help you learn the material you need to know.

3. Subjects were asked to write about _____ events in their lives for _____ consecutive days, especially things they _____. A control group wrote about _____ topics for 4 days. All writing took place in the _____. There was a total of _____ subjects.

4. Dependent variables included self-reported mood _____ and _____ writing, measures of _____ arousal, like blood pressure and heart rate,

and _____ assays of blood before the study, _____ afterwards, and _____ weeks later.

5.   Evaluations by researchers of what the students wrote about confirmed that they had written about _____ experiences, like serious _____ conflict. Immediately after writing, subjects in the experimental group were more _____ than those in the control group. However, they had significantly fewer visits to the _____ and better _____ responses over the next 6 weeks. No differences were found on the measures of _____. If they wrote about previously _____ events they showed better _____ pressure and immunological functioning.

Longitudinal Research Designs: The text discusses this type of research design in the Research Methods section. Finding the answers to these questions will help you get a good understanding of these issues.

6.   The basic goal of a longitudinal study is to determine whether: _____

_____.

7.   Which type of research design is more expensive?   **retrospective   prospective**

Which type is used in this study: a research project measuring Type A behaviour and then recontacting subjects in 5 years to see if those with Type A styles had more heart attacks? _____

8.   Why does a longitudinal design not conclusively prove causality?

_____

Brief Essay

As a final exercise, write out answers to the following brief essay questions. Then compare your answers with the material presented in the text.

     After you have answered these questions, review the "critical thinking" questions that are presented at the end of the text chapter. Answering these questions will help you integrate important issues and themes that have been featured throughout the chapter.

1.   Discuss Holmes and Rahe's Social Re-Adjustment Rating Scale. How do they define a *life change unit*? What could be considered some of the strengths of this scale?

What are some of the criticisms of this scale? How would you change this scale to address some of these criticisms?

2. Briefly discuss Hans Selye's and Walter Cannon's approaches to studying stress. In what ways are they similar? In what ways do they differ?

3. What does the chapter mean when it states that cardiovascular disease (CVD) is a *lifestyle disease*? What are the implications of this? How has health psychology attempted to address this?

ANSWER KEY

Key Terms — Matching #1

1. g	8. r	14. j
2. a	9. b	15. l
3. k	10. p	16. c
4. q	11. d	17. o
5. h	12. m	18. n
6. i	13. s	19. e
7. f		

Names You Should Know

1. b
2. a
3. c

Key Terms — Matching #2

a. 13	f. 4	k. 12	p. 10	u. 20
b. 6	g. 14	l. 18	q. 1	
c. 19	h. 8	m. 11	r. 3	
d. 17	i. 15	n. 2	s. 16	
e. 9	j. 7	o. 5	t. 21	

Key Terms — Matching #3

1. a	6. o	11. h	16. k
2. i	7. m	12. b	17. r
3. d	8. j	13. q	18. e
4. l	9. n	14. c	19. s
5. g	10. f	15. p	

Multiple Choice

1. d	4. c	7. a	10. a	13. c	16. d
2. d	5. a	8. d	11. b	14. c	17. d
3. c	6. a	9. a	12. d	15. a	18. b

Review of Concepts

1. hassles
2. irrelevant; important
3. all illnesses are now seen as psychosomatic
4. stress
5. doesn't account for different ages and backgrounds; includes positive life changes; doesn't consider different meanings for different people
6. alarm, resistance, exhaustion
7. circular
8. maladaptive
9. is
10. Cannon; Selye
11. energy
12. true
13. hostile or negative
14. maladaptive
15. epinephrine and norepinephrine
16. false
17. improves
18. false
19. health behaviors
20. true
21. stress
22. false
23. the ratings were unreliable
24. false
25. false
26. true
27. false
28. Africa
29. women
30. First Nations people
31. false
32. false
33. false
34. it has no symptoms
35. true
36. Eastern Europe
37. men
38. low
39. drinking
40. false
41. rue
42. higher
43. high; low
44. children
45. hostility
46. is
47. weight and salt reduction
48. cognitive therapy; stress management; subsequent MIs

Understanding Research

1. state anxiety; physical danger, social evaluation, daily routine stressors, ambiguous situations; most/82%; state anxiety; type of trait anxiety; type of stressor

2. task-oriented coping; emotion-oriented coping; avoidance-oriented coping; physical illness

3. traumatic; 4; had never told anyone about; trivial; laboratory; 50

4. before; after; autonomic; immunological; immediately; 6

5. upsetting; family; upset; student health center; immune; autonomic arousal; undisclosed; blood

6. hypothesized causes come before their assumed effects; illness causing stress; it is expensive

7. prospective; prospective

8. A third variable could cause both.

CHAPTER 9
PERSONALITY DISORDERS

Chapter Outline

I.   Overview

II. Typical Symptoms and Associated Features
    A. Temperament
    B. Dimensions of Personality
    C. Culture and Personality

III. Classification
    A. Cluster A: Paranoid, Schizoid, and Schizotypal Personality Disorders
    B. Cluster B: Antisocial, Borderline, Histrionic, and Narcissistic Personality Disorders
    C. Cluster C: Avoidant, Dependent, and Obsessive-Compulsive Personality Disorders
    D. A Dimensional Perspective on Classification

IV. Epidemiology
    A. Prevalence in Community and Clinical Samples
    B. Gender Differences
        1. Gender Bias and Diagnosis
    C. Stability Over Time

V.   Schizotypal Personality Disorder (SPD)
    A. Brief Historical Perspective
    B. Clinical Features and Comorbidity
    C. Aetiological Considerations
    D. Treatment

VI. Borderline Personality Disorder (BPD)
    A. Brief Historical Perspective
    B. Clinical Features and Comorbidity
    C. Aetiological Considerations
    D. Treatment

VII. Antisocial Personality Disorder (ASPD)
    A. Brief Historical Perspective
    B. Clinical Features and Comorbidity
        1. Antisocial Behaviour Over the Lifespan
    C. Aetiological Considerations
        1. Biological Factors

Learning Objectives

After reviewing the material presented in this chapter, you should be able to:

1. Appreciate the fact that the behaviour of a person with a personality disorder is ego-syntonic, and understand how that impacts assessment of personality disorder.

2. Define temperament and the broader term, personality, and explain the relevance of these concepts to the study of personality disorders.

3. Classify the personality disorders into the three clusters according to the categories: eccentric, dramatic, and anxious.

4. Provide a basic description of each of the ten DSM-IV personality disorders.

5. Compare and contrast the avoidant personality disorder and the dependent personality disorder.

6. Know the basic prevalence rates for personality disorders in general and which are the most and least common specific personality disorders.

7. Describe the key clinical features of schizotypal personality disorder, borderline personality disorder, and antisocial personality disorder.

8. Compare the treatments of schizotypal, borderline, and antisocial personality disorder patients

9. Consider a dimensional approach to understanding and classifying personality disorders that differs from the DSM-IV categorical approach.

Key Terms — Matching #1

The following terms related to personality disorders are important to know. To test your knowledge, match the following terms with their definitions. Answers are listed at the end of the chapter.

a. Personality
b. Personality disorder
c. Antisocial personality disorder
d. Ego-dystonic
e. Ego-syntonic
f. Narcissistic personality disorder
g. Temperament
h. Neuroticism
i. Extraversion
j. Openness to experience
k. Dependent personality disorder
l. Obsessive-compulsive personality disorder
m. Schizophrenia
n. Schizophrenic phenotype
o. Primary process thinking
p. Splitting
q. Impulse control disorders
r. Intermittent explosive disorder
s. Kleptomania
t. Pyromania

1. ____ characteristic styles of relating to the world; evident in first years of life
2. ____ enduring patterns of perceiving, relating to, and thinking about the environment and oneself, displayed in a wide range of important social and personal contexts
3. ____ the idea that the symptoms of schizotypal personality disorder is seen among people who possess the genotype that makes them vulnerable to schizophrenia
4. ____ out of proportion aggressive behaviours resulting in serious assault or destruction of property
5. ____ stealing objects even though they are not needed or beneficial
6. ____ a dimension of personality describing a person's willingness to consider and explore new ideas, feelings, and activities
7. ____ symptoms that the person is distressed by and uncomfortable with
8. ____ the tendency to see people and events alternatively as all good or all bad
9. ____ disorders characterized by failure to resist a temptation to perform some pleasurable or tension-relieving act that is harmful to self or others
10. ____ where the id relieves tensions by imagining the things it desires
11. ____ a dimension of personality describing a person's activity level, especially interest in interacting with others, and the ease of expressing positive emotions
12. ____ deliberate and purposive fire setting accompanied by fascination with fire and not for personal gain
13. ____ symptoms that are comfortable and acceptable to the person
14. ____ an enduring pattern of dependent and submissive behaviour
15. ____ an enduring pattern of thinking and behaviour characterized by pervasive grandiosity and preoccupation with one's achievements
16. ____ a psychotic disorder characterized by hallucinations and delusions as well as by negative symptoms like flat affect and poverty of speech
17. ____ an enduring pattern of thinking and behaviour characterized by perfectionism and inflexibility
18. ____ a pervasive and persistent disregard for, and frequent violation of, the rights of other people, beginning in childhood or adolescence
19. ____ an enduring pattern of inner experience and behaviour that deviates markedly from the expectations of the person's culture

20. ____ a dimension of personality describing emotional stability, particularly in the expression of anxiety, depression, and anger

Key Terms — Matching #2

The following terms related to personality disorders are important to know. To test your knowledge, match the following terms with their definitions. Answers are listed at the end of the chapter.

1. Agreeableness
2. Conscientiousness
3. Culture
4. Cross-cultural psychology
5. Paranoid personality disorder
6. Schizoid personality disorder
7. Schizotypal personality disorder
8. Borderline personality disorder
9. Histrionic personality disorder
10. Avoidant personality disorder
11. Trichotillomania

12. Pathological gambling
13. Dialectical behaviour therapy (DBT)
14. Psychopathy
15. Adolescence-limited antisocial behaviour
16. Life-course-persistent antisocial behaviour
17. Adoptees
18. Sociotropy

a. ____ an enduring pattern of thinking and behaviour characterized by excessive emotionality and attention seeking
b. ____ the scientific study of ways that human behaviour and mental processes are influenced by social and cultural factors
c. ____ an enduring pattern of thinking and behaviour whose primary feature is a pervasive instability of mood, self-image, and interpersonal relationships
d. ____ another term for antisocial personality disorder
e. ____ the shared way of life of a group of people
f. ____ a common form of social behaviour that is often adaptive and disappears by adulthood
g. ____ people separated from their biological parents at an early age and raised by adoptive parents
h. ____ an enduring pattern of thinking and behaviour characterized by a pervasive tendency to be inappropriately suspicious of motives and behaviours of others
i. ____ an enduring pattern of thinking and behaving characterized by pervasive social discomfort, fear of negative evaluation, and timidity
j. ____ pulling out one's hair, resulting in noticeable hair loss
k. ____ an approach to psychotherapy with borderline patients
l. ____ an enduring pattern of thinking and behaviour characterized by pervasive indifference to interacting with others and a diminished range of emotional experience and expression
m. ____ a dimension of personality describing willingness to cooperate and empathize with others

n. ____ antisocial behaviour that spans a person's life
o. ____ dependent interpersonal relationships that set the stage for later depression
p. ____ a dimension of personality describing the person's persistence in the pursuit of goals, ability to organize activities, and dependability
q. ____ repeated maladaptive gambling despite repeated efforts to stop
r. ____ an enduring pattern of discomfort with other people coupled with peculiar thinking and behaviour, which takes the form of perceptual and cognitive disturbances

Names You Should Know - Matching

The following people have played an important role in research and theory of personality disorders. To test your knowledge, match the following names with the descriptions of their contributions to the study of abnormal psychology. Answers are listed at the end of the chapter.

a. Hervey Cleckley   d. Hagop Akiskal   g. Lee Robins
b. Otto Kernberg   e. John Livesley   h. Marsha Linehan
c. John Gunderson   f. Terrie Moffitt

1. ____ furthered the psychodynamic view of borderline personality disorder by developing reliable, descriptive terms to allow reliable diagnosis
2. ____ advocates a psychodynamic theory of borderline personality disorder focusing on the faulty development of ego structure
3. ____ proposed that there are two forms of antisocial behaviour, transient and nontransient
4. ____ wrote early descriptions of psychopathy
5. ____ argued that borderline personality disorder is not a meaningful diagnostic category but a heterogeneous collection of symptoms that are associated with mild forms of brain dysfunction
6. ____ conducted a longitudinal study showing the stability of antisocial behaviour of boys into adulthood
7. ____ proposed that personality disorders are the result of extreme deviation on normal dimensions of personality and that each of these dimensions is a product of biological predispositions and environmental experiences.
8. ____ developed a promising new approach to psychotherapy with borderline patients which combines cognitive and behavioural strategies with more general principles of supportive psychotherapy.

Review of Concepts — Fill in the Blank and True/False

This section will help focus your studying by testing whether you understand the concepts presented in the text. After you have read and reviewed the material, test your comprehension and memory by filling in the following blanks or circling the right answer. Answers are listed at the end of the chapter.

1. People with personality disorders are especially likely to seek psychological treatment:

    true   false

2. What are some reasons why personality disorders are controversial among professionals? _____

    _____

3. The personality disorders are listed on Axis _____ of a diagnosis.

4. Personality disorders are usually ego -   **syntonic** or **dystonic**

5. What DSM-IV personality disorder is not even included in the International Classification Systems of Diseases (ICD-10) which is primarily used in Europe?

    _____

6. Which of the following is not a dimension of temperament?

    irritability   wealth   activity level   fearfulness

7. Under what circumstances could a difficult temperament be adaptive for an infant?

    _____

8. Cultures differ in displays of _____ and in how much they value individualism versus _____.

9. Typologies of personality are likely to be: **limited to the culture in which they are developed** or **applicable across many different cultures.**

10. The behaviour of people who fit Cluster _____ is typically anxious and fearful.

11. The behaviour of people who fit Cluster _____ is typically odd, eccentric, or asocial.

12. The behaviour of people who fit Cluster _____ is typically dramatic, emotional, or erratic.

13. Only criminals meet the diagnostic requirements for antisocial personality disorder:

    true   false

14. There may be an etiological link between histrionic and _____ personality disorders; both reflect a common, underlying tendency toward lack of inhibition and both form shallow, manipulative relationships with others.

15. One of the advantages of a categorical system over a dimensional system of personality diagnosis is that it provides a more complete description of each person: **true** **false**

16. The DSM-IV uses a **categorical** or **dimensional** system with personality disorders.

17. The overall lifetime prevalence for having any type of personality disorder is:
    1-2% **10-14%** **25-30%** **46-50%**

18. Which personality disorder appears to be the least common?_____

19. Very few people who meet the criteria for one personality disorder also meet the criteria for another personality disorder: **true** **false**

20. Which personality disorder is most likely to be represented in inpatient and outpatient treatment settings? _____

21. Borderline personality disorder is more common among **men** or **women**; antisocial personality disorder is more common among **men** or **women**; and dependent personality disorder is more common among **men** or **women**.

22. Some critics argue that criteria for personality disorders are unfairly biased against traditionally **masculine** or **feminine** traits.

23. People diagnosed with borderline personality disorder as a young adult are **more** or **less** likely to still qualify for the diagnosis in their fifties than people diagnosed with schizotypal or schizoid personality disorders.

24. Research indicates that schizotypal personality disorder is genetically related to schizophrenia: **true** **false**

25. When people with personality disorders appear for psychological treatment, it is usually because _____.

26. Research has shown that low doses of antipsychotic medications are effective in alleviating symptoms of schizotypal personality disorder: **true** **false**

27. The difference between impulsive and compulsive behaviour is that the original goal for impulsive behaviour is to experience _____ while for compulsive behaviour it is to avoid _____.

28. Borderline personality disorder is often comorbid with what Axis I disorder? _____

29. Borderline personality disorder patients have often had problematic relationships with their _____.

30. Patients in dialectical behaviour therapy for borderline personality disorder are less likely to _____.

31. There is no evidence that psychotropic medication is effective for borderline personality disorder: **true** **false**

32. Which personality disorder has been studied the most? _____

33. The DSM-IV category of antisocial personality disorder does not include traits relating to _____ that the Cleckley description included.

34. The expression of antisocial personality is likely to _____ as the person ages.

35. Research indicates that antisocial behaviour is caused by both _____ and _____.

36. In one study of adoptees, being raised in an adverse home environment **did** or **did not** increase the likelihood of antisocial behaviour among children with antisocial biological parents; being raised in an adverse home environment **did** or **did not** increase the likelihood of antisocial behaviour among children with nonantisocial biological parents.

37. Children raised in families with inconsistent or absent _____ were more likely to be antisocial as adults.

38. Children with difficult temperaments due to genetic predisposition to antisocial behaviour may induce their parents to _____.

39. There is research evidence that antisocial people lack_____, an emotion that normal people have.

40. Some researchers argue that lack of _____ and pathological egocentricity are more important than low anxiety in understanding antisocial personality disorder.

41. Research shows that experiencing physical abuse in childhood increases risk for _____ personality disorder in adulthood.

42. Research shows that experiencing sexual abuse in childhood increases risk for _____ personality disorder in adulthood.

43. Several forms of treatment have been shown to be effective with antisocial personality disorder: **true**   **false**

44. Behaviour therapy for antisocial personality disorder can produce   **stable**   or **temporary**   changes in behaviour when the person is closely supervised, and these changes   **do**   or   **do not**   generalize to other situations.

45. Research on psychotherapy with psychopaths suggest that they   **improve** **do not change**   **become worse**   after therapy.

46. People with borderline personality disorder become enraged and manipulative and people with dependent personality disorder become clingy and submissive when threatened with _____.

47. What type of parents are likely to foster dependency in their children?

_____

Multiple Choice Questions

The following multiple choice questions will test your comprehension of the material presented in the chapter. Answers are listed at the end of the chapter.

1) John is always on the lookout for potential harm. He has difficulty trusting anyone, even family members, and is consistently suspicious of their motives. He is over-sensitive to minor events, reading into them ulterior meanings. His manner of relating to people has caused him problems at work and home. What type of personality disorder does John likely have?

   a. schizoid
   b. obsessive-compulsive
   c. antisocial
   d. paranoid

2) The overall lifetime prevalence of personality disorders is approximately:

 a. 5 – 9%   c. 15 – 19%
 b. 10 – 14%   d. 20 – 24%

3) Which is a criterion which is used in DSM-IV to define personality disorders?

 a. the person must be aware of how his or her behaviour is maladaptive
 b. the person's behaviour must be rigid and inflexible
 c. the person's behaviour must cause legal problems
 d. the person's behavioural difficulties must have started in childhood

4) Which of the following statements represents an approach that has been used to conceptualize personality disorders?

 a. they are types of personality styles that are closely associated with specific forms of adult psychopathology
 b. they result from problems in childhood development as conceptualized by psychodynamic theories
 c. they are manifestations of the presence of specific psychological deficits
 d. all of the above

5) The Axis I disorder most often diagnosed with borderline personality disorder is:

 a. depression   c. anxiety
 b. substance abuse   d. sexual dysfunction

6) According to the DSM-IV, an important characteristic of personality disorder is:

 a. they are typically experienced as ego-syntonic
 b. the impairment associated with these disorders is more severe than is found in other forms of mental disorder
 c. there is considerable overlap across diagnostic categories
 d. obsessive-compulsive personality disorder demonstrates the greatest amount of overlap with other personality disorders

7) Research focusing on relationships among personality disorders suggests that:

 a. there is little diagnostic overlap across all personality disorder categories
 b. histrionic personality disorder demonstrates the least amount of diagnostic overlap with other personality disorder categories
 c. there is considerable overlap across diagnostic categories
 d. obsessive-compulsive personality disorder demonstrates the greatest amount of overlap with other personality disorders

8) The most common personality disorder in both inpatient and outpatient settings is:

 a. dependent   c. borderline
 b. antisocial   d. paranoid

9) Which statement is correct regarding treatment of personality disorders?

    a. people with personality disorders benefit most from insight-oriented therapy
    b. people with personality disorders who present for treatment often do so because they have another type of mental disorder such as depression
    c. people with personality disorders benefit most from antipsychotic drugs
    d. people with personality disorders who present for treatment usually remain in treatment until it is completed

10) The Axis I disorder most often diagnosed with antisocial personality disorder is:

    a. dissociative fugue
    b. depression
    c. schizophrenia
    d. substance abuse

11) Which is considered the primary feature of borderline personality disorder?

    a. consistent instability in self-image, mood, and interpersonal relationships
    b. extreme social anxiety
    c. consistent disregard for authority figures
    d. extreme fear of rejection from others

12) About _____ of people with personality disorders do NOT seek treatment.

    a. 40%
    b. 60%
    c. 80%
    d. 95%

13) Sam is definitely a loner. He has no close friends and appears to be indifferent to relationships. Other people would describe Tom as distant and aloof. In addition, Sam reports that he does not feel strongly about anything. He can't think of anything that really makes him excited, but he doesn't get upset or distressed about anything either. Sam might qualify for which of the following personality disorders?

    a. borderline
    b. schizoid
    c. paranoid
    d. narcissistic

14) Which of the following has NOT been a proposed explanation for the aetiology of borderline personality disorder?

    a. early substance abuse
    b. negative consequences resulting from parental loss during childhood
    c. a history of physical and sexual abuse
    d. problematic relationships with parents

15) Personality disorders are listed on which axis of DSM-IV?

    a. I
    b. II
    c. III
    d. IV

16) Which statement regarding gender differences in personality disorders is correct?

    a. antisocial personality disorder is more frequently diagnosed in women
    b. men seek treatment for their personality disorders more often than women
    c. the overall prevalence of personality disorders is about equal in men and women
    d. histrionic personality disorder is more likely to be diagnosed in men

17) Which of the following would NOT be considered a characteristic feature of antisocial personality disorder?

    a. emotional instability   c. deceitfulness
    b. failure to conform to social norms   d. irritability and aggressiveness

18) Mary reports that she feels lonely and isolated. Although she has good relations with family members, she is so afraid of negative criticism from others that she tends to distance herself from relationships. She desperately wants to make friends, but is afraid of being rejected. She constantly watches for even minimal signs of disapproval. Which personality disorder diagnosis is most appropriate for Mary?

    a. schizoid   c. narcissistic
    b. histrionic   d. avoidant

19) An advantage of a dimensional system of classifying personality disorders is:

    a. it eliminates the need for diagnosis
    b. personality disorders are more reliably assessed
    c. it is more useful for those individuals whose symptoms and behaviours fall on the boundaries between different personality disorder diagnoses
    d. it requires less time to arrive at a diagnosis

20) Studies investigating the long-term course of antisocial personality disorder indicate that:

    a. antisocial individuals tend to become more careless as they grow older, resulting in increasing numbers of arrests
    b. antisocial individuals continue their criminal activity well into middle age
    c. antisocial individuals reform their behaviour after several incarcerations
    d. people exhibiting antisocial behaviour tend to "burn out" when they reach middle age

21) According to the five-factor model of personality, the willingness to cooperate and empathize with other people is the trait referred to as:

    a. conscientiousness   c. agreeableness
    b. affiliation   d. cooperativeness

22) Larry has extreme difficulty making decisions on his own. He tends to cling to other people and continually asks them for assistance in making even minor decisions. In addition, he constantly asks for his friends' advice and wants to be reassured about everything, even his ability to be a friend. A possible diagnosis for Larry is:

a. dependent personality disorder
b. avoidant personality disorder
c. narcissistic personality disorder
d. borderline personality disorder

23) Individual psychotherapy with borderline patients can be difficult because:

a. borderline patients frequently cannot afford the cost of such treatment
b. borderline patients are often so transient that it is difficult for them to remain in treatment for more than a brief period of time
c. maintaining the type of concentration necessary for individual therapy is particularly difficult for such patients
d. establishing and maintaining the type of close relationship necessary between therapist and patient is particularly difficult for borderlines

24) The personality disorders listed in DSM-IV are divided into how many clusters?

a. 2
b. 3
c. 4
d. 5

25) Research on the genetics of antisocial personality disorder suggests which of the following statements?

a. genetic and environmental factors combine to produce criminal behaviour
b. the presence of any type of genetic factor in the production of antisocial behaviour is dubious
c. without the presence of genetic factors, environmental factors alone can never predict the development of criminal behaviour
d. environmental factors are much more important than genetic factors in the production of criminal behaviour

26) Sally takes pride in efficient performance and rational behaviour. While others see her as rigid, perfectionistic, inflexible, and judgmental, Sally believes that others simply do not share the same standards and are not worthy of her high opinion. She does not show affection and finds "mushy" feelings in others distasteful. Which personality disorder might Sally have?

a. schizotypal
b. antisocial
c. obsessive-compulsive
d. schizoid

27) Which statement regarding treatment of antisocial personalities is correct?

   a. treatment is usually successful if the individual does not have a history of legal difficulties

   b. currently the best treatment available for this disorder is family therapy

   c. approximately two-thirds of individuals with this disorder show clinical improvement if treated with psychodynamic therapy

   d. the presence of depression in people with this disorder may be associated with a better prognosis for treatment for this disorder

Understanding Research — Fill in the Blank

Canadian Focus: Dimensional Assessment of Personality Pathology: The text presents a detailed description of research by University of British Columbia Psychologist and Psychiatrist, W. John Livesley. Livesley has been primarily interested in understanding the building blocks of personality disorder and the extent to which these traits are influenced by genes and by the environment. Finding the answers to these questions will help you get a good understanding of this area of research and why it is important. It is not necessary to memorize the answers; the process of finding them in the textbook will help you learn the material you need to know.

1.   To identify the important traits involved in personality disorder, Livesley surveyed the scientific literature and the opinions of _____. He and his colleagues performed a statistical technique called _____ to identify the key traits involved in personality disorder. Over a dozen traits were identified which cover _____ of the traits covered in the DSM-IV personality disorders.

2.   These researchers also investigated how these traits group together. The results indicated that traits tended to group together on the following four major dimensions of personality: _____, _____, _____, and _____. These major dimensions were shown to overlap with _____ out of five of the big personality dimensions proposed by the five factor model of normal personality.

3.   Finally, these researchers also investigated the genetic and environmental contribution to these dimensions using a _____ study. They found that there were specific genetic and environmental influences that were _____ to each of

the four dimensions as well as more general environmental factors that were

_____ to all four dimensions.

4.   The significance of Livesley's research is that it emphasizes the idea that personali-

ty disorder consists of _____, not _____. Furthermore, the

results suggest that there is a _____ between normal and abnormal

personality. Finally, the results suggest that many different types of genetic and

environmental influences are at play in the aetiology of personality disorders.

Making Cross-Cultural Comparisons: The text discusses this issue in research in the
Research Methods section. Finding the answers to these questions will help you get a
good understanding of these issues.

5.   What type of subject is the most commonly studied? _____

Who in the United States has been neglected in terms of research?

_____ _____ How are a culture's expectations for behaviour

passed down? _____ Culture shapes people's most basic

view of _____. Among Native Americans, hearing

_____ is a common, normal response.

6.   Researchers interested in cross-cultural comparisons look at differences in the

_____of a disorder in different cultures. They examine how

casual _____may be different. One difficulty in this type of

research is how to determine who shares a _____culture. Another

difficulty is being sure to use comparable _____in the different cul-

tures. _____ the differences that are found is another challenge.

Researchers must also be careful to avoid _____bias in their

interpretations.

Brief Essay

As a final exercise, write out answers to the following brief essay questions. Then compare your answers with the material presented in the text.
    After you have answered these questions, review the "critical thinking" questions
that are presented at the end of the text chapter. Answering these questions will help
you integrate important issues and themes that have been featured throughout the
chapter.

1. Describe the five-factor model of personality. What are the five factors and their definitions? What would be characteristics of low and high scorers on these traits?

2. Discuss the problems associated with the treatment of individuals with personality disorders. Why is a poor prognosis for treatment associated with most of these disorders? What treatment approaches seem most promising to you?

3. Review the controversies that surround the issue of stability of personality. What methods have been used in the attempt to demonstrate stable traits? What do you think are methodological limitations of these approaches?

4. Pretend that you are on the committee to develop DSM-V. Would you recommend classifying personality disorders using a dimensional or categorical approach? Why?

ANSWER KEY

Key Terms

1. g	8. p		
2. a	9. q		
3. n	10. o		
4. r	11. i		
5. s	12. t		
6. j	13. e		
7. d	14. k		

Names You Should Know

1. c	7. e
2. b	8. h
3. f	
4. a	
5. d	
6. g	

Key Terms - Matching #2

a. 9	f. 16	k. 14	p. 19
b. 4	g. 18	l. 6	q. 2
c. 8	h. 5	m. 1	r. 12
d. 15	i. 10	n. 13	s. 7
e. 3	j. 11	o. 17	

Review of Concepts

1. false
2. difficult to diagnose reliably; aetiology is poorly understood; little evidence they are treatable
3. II
4. syntonic
5. narcissistic personality disorder
6. wealth
7. during a famine, while being raised in an institution, in a busy daycare centre
8. emotion, collectivism
9. limited to the culture where it was developed
10. C
11. A

12.	B	31.	true
13.	false	32.	antisocial
14.	antisocial	33.	emotions and interpersonal behaviour
15.	false	34.	change forms
16.	categorical	35.	genes; environment
17.	10-14%	36.	did; did not
18.	narcissistic	37.	discipline
19.	false	38.	be inconsistent or give up in discipline
20.	borderline	39.	fear or anxiety
21.	women; men; women	40.	shame
22.	feminine	41.	antisocial
23.	less	42.	borderline
24.	true	43.	false
25.	have another mental disorder	44.	temporary; do not
26.	true	45.	become worse
27.	pleasure; anxiety	46.	abandonment
28.	depression	47.	overprotective, authoritarian
29.	parents		
30.	leave treatment		

Multiple Choice

1.	d	7.	c	13.	b	19.	c	25.	a
2.	b	8.	c	14.	a	20.	d	26.	c
3.	b	9.	b	15.	b	21.	c	27.	d
4.	d	10.	d	16.	c	22.	a		
5.	a	11.	a	17.	a	23.	d		
6.	a	12.	c	18.	d	24.	b		

Understanding Research

1. experts in personality disorder; factor analysis; most

2. emotional dysregulation; dissocial behaviour; inhibitedness; compulsivity; 4

3. twin; specific; common

4. dimensions; discrete categories; continuum

5. college students in the United States; ethnic minorities; social learning; reality; voices of the dead

6. rates; mechanisms; common; measures; interpreting; cultural

CHAPTER 10
EATING DISORDERS

Chapter Outline

I.   Overview

II. Typical Symptoms and Associated Features of Anorexia Nervosa
- A. Refusal to Maintain a Normal Weight
- B. Disturbance in Evaluating Weight or Shape
- C. Fear of Gaining Weight
- D. Cessation of Menstruation
- E. Medical Complications
- F. Struggle for Control
- G. Comorbid Psychological Disorders

III. Typical Symptoms and Associated Features of Bulimia Nervosa
- A. Binge Eating
- B. Inappropriate Compensatory Behaviour
- C. Excessive Emphasis on Weight and Shape
- D. Comorbid Psychological Disorders
- E. Medical Complications

IV. Classification of Eating Disorders
- A. Brief Historical Perspective
- B. Contemporary Classification
  1. Anorexia Nervosa
  2. Bulimia Nervosa
  3. Binge Eating Disorder and Obesity

V.   Epidemiology of Eating Disorders
- A. Gender Differences and Standards of Beauty
- B. Age of Onset

VI. Aetiological Considerations and Research
- A. Social Factors
  1. Troubled Family Relationships
- B. Psychological Factors
  1. A Struggle for Control
  2. Depression, Low Self-Esteem, and Dysphoria
  3. Negative Body Image
  4. Dietary Restraint

Learning Objectives

After reviewing the material presented in this chapter, you should be able to:

1. Know a basic definition of eating disorders, anorexia nervosa, and bulimia nervosa.

2. Describe the ways in which those with anorexia have distorted perceptions of their weight and shape.

3. Identify the common medical complications associated with anorexia nervosa and bulimia nervosa.

4. Describe some of the typical symptoms of bulimia nervosa, and the inappropriate compensatory behaviour that typifies the disorder.

5. Identify the two subtypes of anorexia nervosa and bulimia nervosa.

6. Know the gender differences involved in eating disorders.

7. Define interoceptive awareness and distorted body image, and understand how they play a role in eating disorders.

8. Identify some of the chief social, psychological, and biological factors responsible for the development of eating disorders.

9. Understand the concept of weight set point.

10. Know the basic goals and techniques utilized in the treatment of anorexia nervosa and bulimia nervosa.

11. Understand the common course and outcome associated with each of these disorders.

Key Terms — Matching

The following terms related to eating disorders are important to know. To test your knowledge, match the following terms with their definitions. Answers are listed at the end of the chapter.

a.   Eating disorders
b.   Anorexia nervosa
c.   Bulimia nervosa
d.   Body mass index
e.   Distorted body image
f.   Amenorrhea
g.   Lanugo
h.   Electrolyte imbalance
i.   Binge eating
j.   Purging
k.   Rumination

l.   Binge eating disorder
m.   Obesity
n.   Incidence
o.   Cohort effects
p.   Enmeshed families
q.   Perfectionism
r.   Introceptive awareness
s.   Effects of dietary restraint
t.   Weight set points
u.   Hypothalamus

1. ____   a fine, downy hair on the face or trunk of the body
2. ____   number of new cases
3. ____   eating an amount of food in a fixed period of time that is clearly larger than most people would eat under similar circumstances
4. ____   the area of the brain that regulates routine biological functions like appetite
5. ____   absence of at least three consecutive menstrual cycles
6. ____   differences that distinguish one group, born during a particular time period, from another group born at a different time period
7. ____   a disturbance in the levels of potassium, sodium, calcium, and other vital elements found in bodily fluids that can lead to cardiac arrest or kidney failure
8. ____   families whose members are overly involved in one another's lives
9. ____   the endless pursuit of unrealistically high standards
10. ____   repeated episodes of binge eating followed by inappropriate compensatory behaviours with other symptoms related to eating and body image
11. ____   excess body fat; body weight over 20 percent above the expected weight
12. ____   an inaccuracy in how one perceives their body size and shape
13. ____   an intentional act designed to eliminate consumed food from the body
14. ____   severe disturbances in eating behaviour that result from fear of gaining weight
15. ____   direct consequences of restricted eating
16. ____   a controversial diagnosis defined by repeated episodes of binge eating in the absence of compensatory behaviour
17. ____   the body's preference for a fixed weight that may have biologically controlled homeostatic mechanisms
18. ____   refusal to maintain a minimally normal body weight along with other symptoms related to eating and body image

19. ____ the regurgitation and rechewing of food
20. ____ recognition of internal cues including emotional states as well as hunger
21. ____ a calculation derived from weight and height used to determine whether someone is significantly underweight

Names You Should Know — Matching

The following people have played an important role in research and theory of eating disorders. To test your knowledge, match the following names with the descriptions of their contributions to the study of abnormal psychology. Answers are listed at the end of the chapter.

a. Hilde Bruch   b. Christopher Fairburn   c. Paul Garfinkel

1. ____ leading researcher of eating disorders, proposed a system for categorizing anorexia nervosa that was incorporated into the DSM-IV classification system.
2. ____ asserted that a struggle for control and perfectionism is the central psychological issue in the development of eating disorders
3. ____ developed a cognitive behavioural treatment for bulimia nervosa

Review of Concepts — Fill in the Blank and True/False

This section will help focus your studying by testing whether you understand the concepts presented in the text. After you have read and reviewed the material, test your comprehension and memory by filling in the following blanks or circling the right answer. Answers are listed at the end of the chapter.

1. People with anorexia nervosa suffer from a loss of appetite: **true   false**

2. Anorexia and bulimia are how much more common in women than in men:

    twice as common   four times as common   ten times as common

3. Males in our society see themselves as thin when they weight 105 percent of their expected weight, while females see themselves as thin when they weight 90 percent of their expected weight: **true   false**

4. Female anorexics are likely to be proud of their emaciation, while male anorexics are likely to be stigmatized for it: **true   false**

5. Eating disorders are more common among men who are wrestlers and men who are gay: **true   false**

6. Often eating disorders begin with a _____.

7. What percent of people admitted to hospitals with anorexia nervosa die of starvation, suicide, or medical complications? _____

8. A person with anorexia often becomes more and more afraid of fat the thinner they become: **true   false**

9. It is likely that amenorrhea and lack of interest in sex common among anorexics are a result rather than a predisposition of the weight loss: **true   false**

10. Although anorexia is a serious mental disorder, it seldom involves medical complications: **true   false**

11. A person with anorexia can be seen as exceptionally successful in what area? _____

12. The study with World War II conscientious objectors found that obsessive-compulsive behaviors probably   **precede**   or   **follow**   the change in eating patterns.

13. Anorexia seldom co-occurs with symptoms of bulimia: **true   false**

14. Binge eating is often triggered by _____.

15. Lack of control is characteristic of _____ while excessive control is characteristic of _____.

16. Vomiting prevents the absorption of how many of the calories consumed during a binge?   **almost none   about half   almost all**

17. The two subtypes of anorexia are the _____ type and the _____ type.

18. The two subtypes of bulimia are the _____ type and the _____ type.

19. Research indicates that obesity is primarily caused by lack of willpower in eating habits: **true   false**

20. Eating disorders have become somewhat less common since the 1960s and 1970s: **true   false**

21. Which type of eating disorder is more common? _____

22. In Third World countries, weighing more is a status symbol: **true**   **false**

23. Studies have shown that physical _____ predicts self-esteem among girls and physical _____predicts self-esteem among boys.

24. People with which type of eating disorder are more likely to report that their families have high levels of conflict? _____

25. Clinicians note that enmeshed families are more characteristic of people with which type of eating disorder? _____

26. Perfectionism is characteristic of people with which type of eating disorder?

    _____

27. Negative evaluations of one's weight, shape, and appearance predict the subsequent development of eating disorders: **true**   **false**

28. There is evidence that diets can be the trigger for the development of an eating disorder: **true**   **false**

29. When food intake is reduced, there is an increase in the metabolic rate:
    true   **false**

30. There is strong evidence that eating disorders are genetic: **true**   **false**

31. There is evidence that family therapy is more effective than individual therapy in treating adolescents with anorexia: **true**   **false**

32. Current forms of treatment for anorexia are quite effective: **true**   **false**

33. Psychotherapy tends to be more effective than antidepressant medication in the treatment of bulimia: **true**   **false**

34. Interpersonal therapy was found to be as effective as cognitive behaviour therapy in the treatment of bulimia: **true**   **false**

35. Bulimia is more likely to lead to death than anorexia: **true**   **false**

Multiple Choice Questions

The following multiple choice questions will test your comprehension of the material presented in the chapter. Answers are listed at the end of the chapter.

1) Both bulimia and anorexia nervosa are characterized by which of the following?

   a. struggle for control
   b. considerable shame

   c. obsessive-compulsive disorder
   d. the absence of menstruation

2) All of the following are compensatory behaviours of bulimia nervosa EXCEPT:

   a. misuse of laxatives
   b. complete avoidance of food

   c. intense exercise
   d. misuse of enemas

3) All of the following are symptoms of anorexia nervosa EXCEPT:

   a. an intense fear of gaining weight
   b. refusal to maintain weight at or above minimally normal weight for age and height
   c. acknowledgment of the seriousness of low body weight, but refusal to change eating behaviour
   d. amenorrhea, or the absence of menstruation

4) Which of the following theories offers the most promising explanations for eating disorders?

   a. biological
   b. social
   c. psychological
   d. all of the above equally offer promising explanations of eating disorders

5) All of the following are symptoms of bulimia nervosa EXCEPT:

   a. recurrent episodes of binge eating that involve large amounts of food
   b. occurs solely during episodes of anorexia nervosa
   c. recurrent inappropriate compensatory behaviour, especially purging
   d. undue influence of weight and body shape on self-evaluation

6) Both bulimia and anorexia nervosa are approximately _____ times more common among women than among men.

   a. 10
   b. 15

   c. 20
   d. 25

7) Many professionals agree that anorexia is a source of which of the following?

   a. shame
   b. pride

   c. gratification
   d. resentment

8) Bulimia nervosa is most prevalent among which of the following groups?

    a. women born after 1960   c. girls ages 10–15
    b. women born before 1950   d. women born in the 1950s

9) Which of the following is NOT a finding that provides evidence that social factors are very important in eating disorders?

    a. eating disorders have recently become much more common
    b. eating disorders are much more common among women working in fields that emphasize weight and appearance, such as modeling and ballet
    c. eating disorders are more common among middle- and upper-class whites
    d. eating disorders have a higher concordance rate in MZ rather than DZ twins

10) Medical complications from anorexia can include all but:

    a. growth of downy hair on the face
    b. dry, cracked skin
    c. hallucinations
    d. kidney failure

Understanding Research — Fill in the Blank

Designing Credible Placebo Control Groups: The test discusses this research issue in the Research Methods section. Finding the answers to these questions will help you get a good understanding of these issues.

1. Which is more difficult, creating a placebo control group for testing a new medication or for testing a new psychological treatment? _____

    _____ Why is this hard? _____

    _____

2. Psychotherapy outcome researchers typically find a treatment that they ally with to be more effective; what is this called? _____ This effect is usually countered with the _____ approach in medication trials, which is impossible to recreate in psychotherapy studies. What is one way to overcome the allegiance effect? _____

    _____

    _____

    What are two problems created by this approach? _____,

    and _____.

Brief Essay

As a final exercise, write out answers to the following brief essay questions. Then compare your answers with the material presented in the text.

After you have answered these questions, review the "critical thinking" questions that are presented at the end of the text chapter. Answering these questions will help you integrate important issues and themes that have been featured throughout the chapter.

1. Discuss the differences between anorexia nervosa and bulimia nervosa in terms of their symptoms, prevalence, aetiology, and treatment.

2. Discuss the evidence that social factors play a role in the aetiology of eating disorders.

3. If you were a therapist and a young woman entered therapy for an eating disorder, what would your treatment plan entail? Would your treatment for a male patient differ from treatment for a female patient? Explain why or why not.

ANSWER KEY

Key Terms — Matching

1. g	8. p	15. s
2. n	9. q	16. l
3. i	10. c	17. t
4. u	11. m	18. b
5. f	12. e	19. k
6. o	13. j	20. r
7. h	14. a	21. d

Names You Should Know

1. c
2. a
3. b

Review of Concepts

1. false	13. false
2. ten times as common	14. an unhappy mood
3. true	15. bulimia; anorexia
4. true	16. about half
5. true	17. restricting; binge-eating/purging
6. diet	18. purging; nonpurging
7. 10 percent	19. false
8. true	20. false
9. true	21. bulimia
10. false	22. true
11. self-control	23. attractiveness; competence
12. follow	24. bulimia

25. anorexia	31. true
26. anorexia	32. false
27. true	33. true
28. true	34. true
29. false	35. false
30. false	

Multiple Choice

1. a	4. b	7. b	10. c
2. b	5. b	8. a	
3. c	6. a	9. d	

Understanding Research

1. testing a new psychological treatment; because developing placebo control for psychological interventions is very difficult.

2. allegiance effect; double-blind; having investigators with opposing allegiances participate in the same study; no placebo control; can't control for differences among therapists

CHAPTER 11
SUBSTANCE USE DISORDERS

Chapter Outline

V. Aetiological Considerations and Research
    A. Social Factors
    B. Biological Factors
        1. Genetics of Alcoholism
            a. Twin Studies
            b. Adoption Studies
        2. Neurochemical Modes of Action
            a. Endogenous Opioid Peptides
            b. The Serotonin Hypothesis
    C. Psychological Factors
        1. Expectations About Drug Effects
        2. Attention Allocation
    D. Integrated Systems

VI. Treatment
    A. Detoxification
    B. Medications during Remission
    C. Self-Help Groups: Alcoholics Anonymous
    D. Cognitive Behaviour Therapy
        1. Coping Skills Training
        2. Relapse Prevention
        3. Short-Term Motivational Therapy
    E. Outcome Results and General Conclusions

Learning Objectives

After reviewing the material presented in this chapter, you should be able to:

1.   Distinguish substance abuse, substance dependence, and polysubstance abuse.

2.   Define tolerance and withdrawal.

3.   Name some of the main short-term effects and consequences of prolonged abuse of alcohol.

4.   Describe some of the properties, short-term effects, and consequences of prolonged use and abuse of the following drugs: barbiturates and benzodiazepines, opiates, nicotine, amphetamines and cocaine, cannabis, and hallucinogens

5.   Know the classification system that DSM-IV uses to differentiate between substance abuse and substance dependence.

6.   Describe the typical course and outcome of alcoholism.

7. Know the epidemiology, including gender differences, of alcoholism and controlled substances.

8. Explain how social factors influence the initial experimentation with drugs and alcohol.

9. State some of the basic findings regarding the genetics of alcoholism—from twin and adoption studies.

10. Explain the endorphin hypothesis and the serotonin hypothesis.

11. Understand the importance of cognitive expectations in the effects of alcohol.

12. Delineate the attention allocation model and how it explains the typical functioning of inebriated people.

13. Understand the integrated systems approach to substance use and abuse.

14. Describe the following treatment programs: detoxification, self-help groups, controlled drinking training, and relapse prevention training.

15. Review the research exploring the effectiveness of matching clients to different types of treatments for addiction.

Key Terms — Matching #1

The following terms related to substance use disorders are important to know. To test your knowledge, match the following terms with their definitions. Answers are listed at the end of the chapter.

a.	Substance dependence	n.	Alcohol withdrawal delirium
b.	Substance abuse	o.	Delirium tremens
c.	Polysubstance abuse	p.	Tranquilizers
d.	Addiction	q.	Barbiturates
e.	Psychoactive substance	r.	Benzodiazepines
f.	Hypnotics	s.	Cocaine
g.	Sedatives (anxiolytic)	t.	Opiates
h.	Narcotic analgesics	u.	Morphine
i.	Craving	v.	Codeine
j.	Psychological dependence	w.	Heroin
k.	Physiological dependence	x.	Methadone
l.	Tolerance	y.	Psychomotor stimulants
m.	Withdrawal		

1. ____ CNS depressants that are used for relieving anxiety
2. ____ a less severe pattern of drug use defined in terms of interference with a person's ability to fulfill major role obligations, the recurrent use of a drug in dangerous situations, or the experience of legal problems associated with the drug use
3. ____ drugs with properties similar to opium, often used to relieve pain
4. ____ convulsions, hallucinations, and a sudden disturbance of consciousness with changes in cognitive processes during withdrawal from alcohol
5. ____ the process through which the nervous system becomes less sensitive to the effects of a substance with repeated exposure to that substance
6. ____ a synthetic opiate often injected, inhaled, or smoked
7. ____ physical symptoms related to drug use, including tolerance and withdrawal
8. ____ a class of drugs, discovered in the early twentieth century, used widely for many years to treat anxiety, prevent seizures, and relieve pain
9. ____ drugs which produce their effects by simulating the actions of certain neurotransmitters
10. ____ also known as drug of abuse; a chemical substance that alters mood, level of perception, or brain functioning
11. ____ a synthetic opiate sometimes used therapeutically as an alternative to heroin
12. ____ used to decrease anxiety or agitation
13. ____ CNS depressants that are used to help people sleep
14. ____ the abuse of several types of drugs
15. ____ opiates that can be used clinically to decrease pain
16. ____ a forceful urge to use drugs
17. ____ symptoms experienced when a person stops using a drug
18. ____ a more severe pattern of repeated self-administration often resulting in tolerance, withdrawal, or compulsive drug-taking behaviour
19. ____ one of the active ingredients of opium, very similar to heroin
20. ____ one of the active ingredients of opium, available in small quantities in Canada in over-the-counter medications
21. ____ an older term used to describe substance use problems such as alcoholism
22. ____ feeling compelled to use a drug to control one's feelings or to prepare for certain activities
23. ____ an older term for alcohol withdrawal delirium
24. ____ synthetic drugs whose therapeutic effects were discovered in the 1950s which have largely replaced barbiturates in medical practice
25. ____ a naturally occurring stimulant drug extracted from the leaf of a small tree that grows at high elevations

Key Terms — Matching #2

The following terms related to substance use disorders are important to know. To test your knowledge, match the following terms with their definitions. Answers are listed at the end of the chapter.

1. Amphetamines
2. Naltrexone
3. Amphetamine psychosis
4. Cannabis
5. Marijuana
6. Hashish
7. Temporal disintegration
8. Reverse tolerance
9. Hallucinogens
10. LSD
11. Psilocybin
12. Mescaline
13. Peyote
14. Pencyclidine (PCP)
15. Acamprosate
16. Flashbacks
17. Endorphins
18. Balanced placebo design
19. Risk
20. Relative risk
21. High-risk research design
22. Vulnerability indicators
23. Alcohol myopia
24. Detoxification
25. Antabuse
26. Abstinence violation effect

a. _____ the dried leaves and flowers of the hemp plant

b. _____ a medication used in Europe to treat alcoholism; not yet approved by the FDA

c. _____ a newly approved medication to treat alcoholism which has been demonstrated to be effective in reducing relapse rates

d. _____ synthetically produced psychomotor stimulants such as dexedrine or methamphetamine

e. _____ a procedure that allows the investigator to separate the direct, biological effects of the drug from the subjects' expectations about how the drug should affect their behaviour

f. _____ drugs that cause people to experience hallucinations at relatively low doses

g. _____ a drug that can block the chemical breakdown of alcohol which will make the person taking it violently ill if he or she consumes alcohol

h. _____ brief visual after effects that can occur at unpredictable intervals long after a hallucinogen has cleared the body

i. _____ a technique where subjects are selected from the general population based on some identified risk factor that has a fairly high risk ratio

j. _____ auditory or visual hallucinations as well as delusions of persecution or grandeur that can occur with high doses of amphetamines or cocaine and usually disappears after the drug is metabolized

k. _____ manifestations of the genotype associated with a mental disorder

l. _____ a hallucinogen found in certain mushrooms which bears a chemical resemblance to serotonin

m. _____ a synthetic hallucinogen that bears a strong chemical resemblance to serotonin

n. _____ a condition often accompanying cannabis intoxication in which people have trouble retaining and organizing information

o. _____ becoming more sensitive to a drug with prolonged use; reported by users but not yet documented in laboratory studies

p.	____	a synthetic drug that can induce psychotic behaviour at high doses
q.	____	the probability that a certain outcome will occur
r.	____	the probability that someone with a certain characteristic will develop a disorder divided by the probability that someone without the same characteristic will develop the same disorder
s.	____	the guilt and perceived loss of control that a person feels whenever he or she slips and takes a drug after an extended period of abstinence
t.	____	the removal of a drug on which a person has become dependent
u.	____	a drug with the active ingredient called THC, derived from the hemp plant
v.	____	a type of hallucinogen that resembles norepinephrine
w.	____	the dried resin from the top of the female hemp plant
x.	____	a marked tendency to engage in shortsighted information processing when intoxicated
y.	____	a cactus that contains mescaline
z.	____	endogenous opioids that are naturally synthesized in the brain and are closely related to morphine

Names You Should Know — Matching

The following people have played an important role in research and theory of substance use disorders. To test your knowledge, match the following names with the descriptions of their contributions to the study of abnormal psychology. Answers are listed at the end of the chapter.

a. George Vaillant
b. Alan Marlatt
c. Linda and Mark Sobell

d. Robert Cloninger
e. Robert Pihl

1. ____ proposed that there were two types of alcoholism, Type I, which has a later onset, psychological dependence, and the absence of antisocial personality traits, and Type II, which is predominantly among men, has an earlier onset, and co-occurs with antisocial behaviours

2. ____ conducted a longitudinal study of alcoholism among inner-city adolescents and college students

3. ____ developed a cognitive behavioural view of the relapse process and a relapse prevention model for treatment of substance use.

4. ____ researchers who advocated and then provided empirical support for the "controlled drinking" approach to alcoholism treatment which strongly challenged the disease model of alcoholism.

5. ____ a researcher whose experimental studies have greatly contributed to the understanding of the many variables influencing drinking behaviour

Review of Concepts — Fill in the Blank and True/False

This section will help focus your studying by testing whether you understand the concepts presented in the text. After you have read and reviewed the material, test your comprehension and memory by filling in the following blanks or circling the right answer. Answers are listed at the end of the chapter.

1. Most researchers have moved toward a view of substance abuse that emphasizes common causes, behaviours, and consequences of using the substance rather than a focus on the particular drug used: **true   false**

2. One of the best indices for defining alcoholism is the amount of alcohol a person consumes: **true   false**

3. A crucial feature of alcoholism is diminished _____.

4. The most substantial tolerance effects are found among people who use which drugs? _____
    _____

5. What drugs have not been shown to have tolerance effects? _____

6. _____is the most widely used psychoactive substance in the world.

7. What organ metabolizes alcohol? _____

8. Blood alcohol levels are only weakly correlated with intoxicating effects:
    true   false

9. When blood alcohol levels go too high, the person will become unconscious and can always sleep off the effects of the alcohol with no acute dangers:
    true   false

10. There is a strong correlation between crime and alcohol: **true   false**

11. The abuse of alcohol has more negative health consequences over an extended period of time than any other drug: **true   false**

12. Sedatives and hypnotics can lead to a state of arousal similar to that of cocaine:
    true   false

13. When used to reduce anxiety, barbiturates and benzodiazepines produce a calm, relaxed feeling: **true**   **false**

14. Barbiturates may not be helpful because a return in symptoms occurs when a person stops taking them: **true**   **false**

15. Opiates produce what kind of subjective effect? _____.

16. Heroin addicts suffer from few health problems and are not more likely to die than non-addicts.   **true**   **false**

17. Nicotine may mimic the effects of _____ drugs.

18. Nicotine produces CNS   **arousal**   or   **depression.**

19. Babies born to mothers who smoked during pregnancy weigh   **more**   or   **less** than those born to mothers who did not smoke.

20. At what age does addiction to nicotine almost always begin? _____

21. From a psychological point of view, withdrawal from nicotine is just as difficult as withdrawal from _____.

22. Cocaine and amphetamines activate the sympathetic nervous system:
    true   **false**

23. Amphetamine psychosis is a permanent condition: **true**   **false**

24. The most common reaction to discontinuing stimulant drugs is _____

25. Marijuana and hashish show strong tolerance effects: **true**   **false**

26. Hallucinogens may trigger persistent psychosis is people vulnerable to that type of disorder: **true**   **false**

27. Culture, not the nature of the drug, shapes people's choices about drug use and the ways in which they use them: **true**   **false**

28. Most alcoholics go through repeated periods of _____.

29. In Vaillant's study, relapse to alcohol abuse was unlikely if the period of abstinence- was how many years? _____

30. What three types of disorders are commonly associated with alcohol abuse?

_____, _____, and

_____.

31. Cannabis is used almost exclusively in North America: **true   false**

32. Among all men and women who have ever used alcohol, about _____ percent will develop serious problems with drinking sometime during their lives.

33. Men outnumber women in chronic abuse of alcohol by a ratio of about:

3 to 1   5 to 1   10 to 1

34. Women who drink experience more social _____ than men.

35. Women metabolize alcohol more slowly than men, even when differences in body weight are controlled: **true   false**

36. The lifetime prevalence for addiction to nicotine is:

4 percent   14 percent   254 percent

37. Nicotine is one of the most addictive drugs in our society   **true   false**

38. The elderly are more likely to be addicted to alcohol than are younger people:

true   false

39. Parents have a greater influence over their children's decision to use _____ and peers seem to play a more important role in the decision to use

_____.

40. Adolescents with alcoholic parents are less likely to drink than those whose parents are not alcoholic: **true   false**

41. A flushing response to even a small amount of alcohol, including flushed skin, nausea, and an abnormal heartbeat occurs in 30-50 percent of people of what ethnic ancestry? _____

42. There is an elevated risk for alcoholism among first-degree relatives of alcoholics:

true   false

43. Twin studies indicate that genetic factors alone are responsible for the increased risk for alcoholism among relatives of alcoholics: **true   false**

44. The Indians of South American who produce coca leaves to sell typically have severe dependence problems: **true   false**

45. Rates of cigarette smoking among young adults declined over the 1990's:
    true   false

46. There is evidence that a deficiency in the activity of what type of neurotransmitter is related to vulnerability to alcoholism? _____

47. The tension-reduction hypothesis suggests that people drink alcohol in an effort to reduce the impact of a _____ environment.

48. In one study, people who believed they consumed alcohol but really did not showed increased _____ and _____ arousal.

49. _____ expectancies about effects of alcohol predict drinking problems.

50. Detoxification from alcohol is typically accomplished by abruptly discontinuing consumption of alcohol: **true   false**

51. Many patients using Antabuse have poor compliance with treatment, that is they stop taking the Antabuse: **true   false**

52. There is no research evidence that Alcoholics Anonymous is an effective form of treatment: **true   false**

53. The heritability estimates for men and women in risk for alcoholism due to genetic factors are about: **1/10   2/3   9/10**

54. The relapse prevention model of treatment teaches patients to interpret slips in abstinence as _____.

55. The results from Project MATCH which compared twelve-step facilitation therapy, relapse prevention and short term motivational enhancement therapy suggest that _____ therapy is preferred over other treatments.

56. The medication _____ works by making a person feel sick if they drink, and the medication _____ works by reducing the rewarding effects of alcohol.

57. Motivational interviewing takes a **confrontational** **nonconfrontational** approach.

58. Research by Conrod, et al., provides support for client-treatment matching for addictive behaviour if the matching strategy targets different

    _____.

Multiple Choice Questions

The following multiple choice questions will test your comprehension of the material presented in the chapter. Answers are listed at the end of the chapter.

1) The two terms included in the DSM-IV to describe substance use disorders are:
   a. substance dependence and substance abuse
   b. substance abuse and addiction
   c. tolerance and addiction
   d. substance abuse and polysubstance abuse

2) Although disulfiram (Antabuse) can effectively block the chemical breakdown of alcohol, people resist using this drug because:
   a. it is an extremely expensive drug to administer
   b. the effect of the drug is very short-lived; that is, it reduces alcohol intake for only a few hours after its ingestion
   c. individuals who use this drug have to monitor their dietary intake
   d. use of the drug produces a dramatically adverse physical reaction

3) Because alcoholism is associated with many diverse problems, distinguishing between people who are dependent on alcohol and those who are not is often determined by which of the following?
   a. the presence of legal problems (e.g., driving under the influence)
   b. whether or not the person reports tolerance to alcohol
   c. the number of problems that the person experiences
   d. the presence of medical problems

4) Research on the long term course of alcohol suggests that:
   a. the typical individual is able to successfully stop drinking only after hospitalization
   b. the typical individual cycles through periods of alcohol consumption, cessation, and relapse
   c. the typical individual rarely experiences relapse after making the decision to stop drinking
   d. the typical individual spends approximately 10 years in the alcohol consumption period before making the decision to quit

5) Which of the following is an example of a CNS stimulant?

    a. alcohol   c. morphine
    b. cocaine   d. hashish

6) Results from adoption studies focusing on the genetic transmission of alcohol indicate that:

    a. the familial nature of alcoholism appears to be at least partially determined by genes; that is, having an alcoholic biological parent increases risk for alcoholism
    b. if a person does not have a alcoholic biological parent, having an adopted parent with alcohol problems greatly increases risk for alcoholism
    c. having the personality trait of "behavioural overcontrol" increases risk for alcoholism
    d. only people with at least one alcoholic biological parent are at risk for alcoholism

7) John currently drinks large amounts of alcohol on a daily basis. He plans his day around when alcohol will be available to him. He drives a certain route home from work that passes two liquor stores to ensure that liquor will be available each evening. His weekend activities are planned around availability of alcohol, and he will not attend social functions where alcohol is absent. Which term best describes his condition?

    a. binge drinker   c. psychological dependence
    b. controlled drinker   d. prealcoholic drinker

8) Although there is much individual variability in how people respond to alcohol, generally, the intoxicating effects of alcohol can be observed (and felt) at blood alcohol concentrations ranging between:

    a. 10-30 mg percent   c. 300-400 mg percent
    b. 150-300 mg percent   d. 400-500 mg percent

9) A person who has a compelling need to use a drug and cannot control or regulate his/her drug use is commonly described as:

    a. in withdrawal   c. intoxicated
    b. a recreational drug user   d. addicted

10) One reason that risk for substance dependence is increased in elderly people is:

    a. the elderly demonstrate a reduced sensitivity to drug toxicity and therefore require higher drug dosages
    b. adult children often encourage their elderly parents to use drugs to control their nerves
    c. the elderly use prescribed psychoactive drugs more frequently than compared to other age groups
    d. in fact, there is little risk for substance dependence in the elderly (less than 1 percent of the population)

11) A principal assumption of Alcoholics Anonymous (AA) is:

  a. people need to relapse several times before they will learn to take their alcohol problem seriously
  b. individuals cannot recover on their own
  c. individuals need to remove themselves from the stressful situations that trigger alcohol use
  d. with enough help, people can develop effective methods of controlled drinking

12) Which of the following statements is accurate regarding the definition of substance dependence in the DSM-IV?

  a. evidence of tolerance and withdrawal is required
  b. the individual must exhibit several characteristics that describe a pattern of compulsive use
  c. the person must exhibit characteristics of problematic substance use for at least two years
  d. a prior diagnosis of substance abuse is required before the diagnosis of substance dependence may be considered

13) Which would NOT be considered an example of a common alcohol expectancy?

  a. alcohol decreases power and aggression
  b. alcohol enhances social and physical pleasure
  c. alcohol enhances sexual performance
  d. alcohol increases social assertiveness

14) Aerosol spray, glue, and paint thinner are all examples of which class of psychoactive drugs?

  a. CNS depressants
  b. over-the-counter drugs
  c. solvents
  d. hallucinogens

15) What percentage of people develop serious problems resulting from prolonged alcohol consumption?

  a. 10 percent
  b. 20 percent
  c. 30 percent
  d. 40 percent

16) Which of the following statements is TRUE regarding alcohol expectancies?

  a. negative expectancies appear to be less powerful than positive expectancies in influencing alcohol use
  b. adolescents do not appear to have strong beliefs about alcohol prior to taking their first drink
  c. expectations regarding alcohol do not predict drinking behaviours
  d. portrayal of alcohol in the mass media does not appear to influence individuals' alcohol expectancies

17) Which of the following statements regarding tolerance is TRUE?

   a. individuals can develop tolerance to all psychoactive drugs over time
   b. certain hallucinogens may not lead to the development of tolerance
   c. the most substantial tolerance effects are found among cannabis users
   d. heroin and CNS stimulants do not lead to the development of tolerance

18) Rates of alcohol abuse are significantly lower among:

   a. Jews
   b. Catholics
   c. Native Americans
   d. Protestants

19) Which of the following statements is TRUE regarding the presence of alcohol dependence over a long period of time?

   a. alcohol dependence always results in Korsakoff's psychosis
   b. alcohol dependence follows opiate dependence and cocaine dependence in terms of potential negative health consequences
   c. nutritional disturbances caused by alcohol dependence can be controlled through appropriate medication
   d. alcohol dependence has more negative health consequences than does abuse of any other substance

20) Which of the following symptoms are side effects of alcohol withdrawal?

   a. hand tremors, sweating, and nausea
   b. anxiety and insomnia
   c. convulsions and hallucinations
   d. all of the above

21) The most promising neurochemical explanation of alcoholism currently focuses on which of the following neurotransmitters?

   a. serotonin   c. epinephrine
   b. dopamine   d. norepinephrine

22) Considering all the direct and indirect ways that alcohol use contributes to death (e.g., suicides, accidents, medical disorders), alcohol is considered:

   a. the first leading cause of death in this country
   b. the second leading cause of death in this country
   c. the third leading cause of death in this country
   d. the fourth leading cause of death in this country

23) Which of the following statements reflects a difference between men and women in their use of alcohol?

    a. the average age of onset for alcoholism is higher among men
    b. women are less likely to develop hepatic disorders even after drinking heavily for many years
    c. women are more likely to report additional symptoms of depression and anxiety, while antisocial personality traits are more likely to be displayed in men
    d. men are more likely to drink if their partners drink

24) Which class of drugs is LEAST associated with severe withdrawal effects?

    a. stimulants
    b. alcohol
    c. sedatives and anxiolytics
    d. opiates

25) One reason that it is difficult to gather epidemiological information on substance use is that:

    a. the definition of substance abuse and dependence has been clearly restricted in the past
    b. this type of research is expensive and therefore has not been adequately funded
    c. drug users are often reluctant to accurately report their drug use because of the illegal status of many drugs
    d. all of the above

Understanding Research — Fill in the Blank

The Swedish Adoption Studies: The text presents a detailed description of a study by Cloninger, Bohman, and Sigvardsson in the Research Close-Up. Finding the answers to these questions will help you get a good understanding of this study and why it is important. It is not necessary to memorize the answers; the process of finding them in the textbook will help you learn the material you need to know.

1.   What are the two types of alcoholism that were evaluated in this study?

    _____ and _____. What were the two cities where subjects were

    collected? _____ and _____. Did the findings from the

    two sites agree? _____ How old were the men at the time of the study?

    Between the ages of _____ and _____. How were these men selected?

    _____

    _____

2.   The information was gathered from the records of local _____

    boards, hospital and _____ records, and the national

_____ register. It was felt that this approach would identify _____ percent of those who had a serious drinking problem. What two types of background were evaluated? _____ and _____.

Which type of alcoholism is characterized by criminal activity and an early age of onset? Type _____.

3. For those with a genetic background of Type 1 alcoholism, a significant increase in the risk of alcoholism was evident in those people with what type of genetic and environmental background? _____

_____.

For those with a genetic background of Type 2 alcoholism, which was a stronger predictor of alcoholism, environmental factors or genetic factors?

_____ Females with a genetic predisposition to Type 1 alcoholism were _____ times more likely to abuse alcohol. Females with a genetic predisposition to Type 2 alcoholism were _____ more likely to abuse alcohol. What is one criticism of this study? _____

_____.

Risk, Risk Factors, and Studies of High-Risk Samples: The text discusses this type of research in the Research Methods section. Finding the answers to these questions will help you get a good understanding of these issues.

4. What is the risk that a person in Canada will develop alcoholism at some point in their lives? _____ What is the risk for all other types of illegal and controlled substances? _____ Risk implies _____, not certainty. What does a relative risk of 3 mean? _____

_____

5. Does risk imply causality? _____ What benefit do longitudinal studies of risk provide? _____

Why aren't they used all the time? _____

What is one technique used to increase the productivity of longitudinal research?

_____ How are subjects selected for this type of research?_____

What is a vulnerability indicator? _____

_____

Brief Essay

As a final exercise, write out answers to the following brief essay questions. Then compare your answers with the material presented in the text.

   After you have answered these questions, review the "critical thinking" questions that are presented at the end of the text chapter. Answering these questions will help you integrate important issues and themes that have been featured throughout the chapter.

1.   Explain Robert Cloniger and Michael Bohman's theory of Type 1 and Type 2 alcoholism. What do you think are possible weaknesses of their model? What further type of research is necessary to support or disconfirm such a theory?

2.   Describe the balanced placebo design. Why is it a useful research design for the study of the effects of alcohol on behaviour?

3.   Review the attention-allocation model of alcohol as proposed by Claude Steele and Robert Josephs. What are the two general factors on which this model is based? How does the theory predict such behaviours as drunken excess, drunken self-inflation, and drunken relief?

4.   Explain why the findings from Sobell and Sobell's (1978) controlled drinking research were met with such skepticism. What implications did their findings have for models of alcoholism that were widely accepted at that time? What current model and treatment approaches are based on the Sobell's controlled drinking research?

ANSWER KEY

Key Terms — Matching #1

1. g	8. q	15. h	22. j
2. b	9. y	16. c	23. o
3. t	10. e	17. m	24. r
4. n	11. x	18. a	25. s
5. l	12. p	19. u	
6. w	13. f	20. v	
7. k	14. c	21. d	

Names You Should Know

1. d
2. a
3. b
4. c
5. e

Key Terms — Matching #2

a. 5	e. 18	i. 21	m. 10	q. 19	u. 4	y. 13
b. 15	f. 9	j. 3	n. 7	r. 20	v. 12	z. 17
c. 2	g. 25	k. 22	o. 8	s. 26	w. 6	
d. 1	h. 16	l. 11	p. 14	t. 24	x. 23	

Review of Concepts

1. true
2. false
3. control over drinking
4. alcohol, nicotine, heroin, cocaine, amphetamines
5. hallucinogens
6. caffeine
7. the liver
8. false
9. false
10. true
11. true
12. false
13. true
14. true
15. euphoria
16. false
17. antidepressant
18. arousal
19. medical device
20. adolescence
21. heroin
22. true
23. false
24. depression
25. false
26. true
27. true
28. abstinence
29. six
30. antisocial personality disorder, mood disorder, and anxiety disorder
31. false
32. 20 percent
33. 5 to 1
34. disapproval
35. true
36. 25 percent
37. true
38. false
39. alcohol; marijuana
40. false
41. Asian
42. true
43. false
44. false
45. false
46. serotonin
47. stressful
48. aggression; sexual
49. positive
50. false
51. true
52. false
53. 2/3
54. temporary
55. no one
56. Antabuse; Naltrexone
57. nonconfrontational
58. personality profiles

195

Multiple Choice

1. a	6. a	11. b	16. a	21. a
2. d	7. c	12. b	17. b	22. d
3. c	8. b	13. a	18. a	23. c
4. b	9. d	14. c	19. d	24. a
5. b	10. c	15. b	20. d	25. c

Understanding Research

1. Type 1; Type 2; Stockholm; Gothenburg; yes; 23; 43; They were born out of wedlock and adopted away at a young age.

2. temperance; insurance; criminal; 70; genetic; environmental; two

3. Both genetic and environmental predispositions to alcoholism were necessary; genetic; three; were not; the measure of environmental factors was limited to social class, which is a crude measure

4. 14 in 10; 8 in 100; probability; the risk for a person with that characteristic is three times higher than the risk for a person without that characteristic

5. No; They can determine causality; They are expensive and time-consuming; High-risk research design; by a risk factor with a high risk ratio; manifestation of the genotype associated with a mental disorder in the absence of the full- blown disorder

CHAPTER 12
SEXUAL AND GENDER IDENTITY DISORDERS

Chapter Outline

   1. Biological Factors
   2. Social Factors
   3. Psychological Factors
  E. Treatment
   1. Aversion Therapy
   2. Cognitive-Behavioural Treatment
   3. Hormones and Medication

IV. Gender Identity Disorders
  A. Typical Symptoms and Associated Features
  B. Epidemiology
  C. Aetiology
  D. Treatment

Learning Objectives

After reviewing the material presented in this chapter, you should be able to:

1. Understand that a great deal of our thinking about sexual disorders is a result of cultural and religious values.

2. Know the role of Freud, Ellis, Kinsey, and Masters and Johnson in the study of human sexuality.

3. Distinguish hypoactive sexual desire from sexual aversion disorder.

4. Define male erectile disorder, female arousal disorder, premature ejaculation, dyspareunia, and female orgasmic disorder.

5. Know which sexual disorders are the most common.

6. List some of the biological and psychological causes of hypoactive sexual desire, disorder of sexual arousal, premature ejaculation, and inhibited orgasm.

7. Describe sensate focus as a treatment technique for sexual disorders.

8. Identify the major forms of paraphilias.

9. Describe some of the causes of paraphilias, including faulty lovemaps, imprinting, courtship disorders, and intimacy deficits.

10. Distinguish disorders of gender identity from disorders of sexual disorder (e.g., transvestic fetishism).

Key Terms — Matching #1

The following terms related to sexal and gender identity disorders are important to know. To test your knowledge, match the following terms with their definitions. Answers are listed at the end of the chapter.

a. Sexual dysfunctions
b. Paraphilias
c. Gender identity
d. Gender identity disorder
e. Excitement
f. Orgasm
g. Resolution
h. Refractory period
i. Probability sampling
j. Convenience sampling

k. Hypoactive sexual desire disorder
l. Sexual aversion disorder
m. Erectile dysfunction
n. Impotence
o. Female sexual arousal disorder
p. Male erectile disorder
q. Inhibited sexual arousal
r. Hypothetical construct
s. Operational definition

1. ____ sudden intensely pleasurable release of sexual tension
2. ____ a strong and persistent identification with the opposite sex coupled with a sense of discomfort with one's anatomical sex
3. ____ a disorder in which a person has an extreme aversion to and avoidance of genital sexual contact with a partner
4. ____ persistent or recurrent erectile dysfunction
5. ____ sampling in which every member of a clearly specified population has a known probability of selection
6. ____ forms of sexual disorder that involve inhibitions of sexual desire or interference with the physiological responses leading to orgasm
7. ____ a procedure used to measure a theoretical construct
8. ____ sampling from a readily available group of participants
9. ____ forms of sexual disorder that involve sexual arousal in association with unusual objects and situations
10. ____ persistent or recurrent inability to attain or maintain an adequate lubrication-swelling response of sexual excitement even in the presence of sexual desire
11. ____ a person's sense of being male or female
12. ____ third stage of Masters and Johnson's human sexual response cycle where the body returns to its resting state
13. ____ disorder characterised by diminished desire for sexual activity and reduced frequency of sexual fantasies
14. ____ first stage of Masters and Johnson's human sexual response cycle involving physiological responses and subjective feelings
15. ____ inability to attain or maintain an adequate lubrication-swelling response of sexual excitement
16. ____ an older term for erectile dysfunction that is no longer used because of its negative implications

17. ____ events or states that reside within a person and are proposed to explain that person's behaviour
18. ____ difficulty in obtaining an erection that is sufficient to accomplish intercourse or to satisfy self or partner during intercourse
19. ____ period of time after orgasm the person is unresponsive to further sexual stimulation

Key Terms — Matching #2

The following terms related to sexual and gender identity disorders are important to know. To test your knowledge, match the following terms with their definitions. Answers are listed at the end of the chapter.

1. Penile plethysmograph
2. Vaginal photometer
3. Construct validity
4. Premature ejaculation
5. Female orgasmic disorder
6. Genital anesthesia
7. Dyspareunia
8. Vaginismus
9. Excessive sexual drive
10. Performance anxiety
11. Sensate focus
12. Scheduling
13. Fetishism
14. Partialism
15. Transvestite
16. Transvestic fetishism
17. Drag queens
18. Transvestic fetishism with gender dysphoria
19. Sexual masochism
20. Sexual sadism

a. ____ the extent that a measure produces results consistent with the theoretical construct it is purported to assess
b. ____ a procedure for measuring male sexual arousal and their erotic preferences
c. ____ a diagnosis included in the ICD but not the DSM
d. ____ a person who dresses in the clothing of the other gender
e. ____ a paraphilia in which sexual arousal is associated with the actual act of being humiliated, beaten, bound, or otherwise made to suffer
f. ____ cross-dressing for sexual arousal with eventual persistent discomfort with gender identity
g. ____ involuntary muscular spasm preventing sexual intercourse
h. ____ setting aside specific time for sexual activity
i. ____ a treatment for sexual dysfunction that involves a series of simple exercises in which the couple spends time in a quiet, relaxed setting, learning to touch each other
j. ____ a paraphilia in which sexual arousal is associated with desires to inflict physical or psychological suffering or humiliation on another person
k. ____ absence of genital sensations during sexual activity
l. ____ a procedure for measuring female sexual arousal
m. ____ association of sexual arousal with nonliving objects

n.   ____   persistent genital pain during or after intercourse

o.   ____   gay men who engage in cross-dressing for reasons other than sexual arousal

p.   ____   inability to achieve orgasm even though a person experiences uninhibited sexual arousal

q.   ____   intense sexual attraction to specific, nonsexual body parts

r.   ____   fear of failure

s.   ____   cross-dressing for the purpose of sexual arousal

t.   ____   a disorder in which a man is unable to delay ejaculation long enough to accomplish intercourse

Key Terms - Matching #3

The following terms related to sexual and gender identity disorders are important to know. To test your knowledge, match the following terms with their definitions. Answers are listed at the end of the chapter.

a. Exhibitionism	k. Opportunistic rapists
b. Voyeurism	l. Lovemap
c. Frotteurism	m. Aversion therapy
d. Pedophilia	n. Community notification laws
e. Incest	o. Sexual predator laws
f. Rape	p. Sex roles
g. Acquaintance rape	q. Transexualism (gender dysphoria)
h. Sadistic rapists	r. Pseudohermaphroditism
i. Nonsadistic rapists	s. Sex-reassignment surgery
j. Vindictive rapists	

1.   ____   a paraphilia characterised by distress over, or acting on, urges to expose one's genitals to an unsuspecting stranger

2.   ____   rape committed by someone known to the victim

3.   ____   sexual activity between close blood relatives (or between stepparents and stepchildren)

4.   ____   a category of rapist who is preoccupied with sadistic sexual fantasies whose actions are brutal and violent

5.   ____   a paraphilia characterised by distress over or acting on urges involving sexual activity with a prepubescent child

6.   ____   discomfort with one's anatomical sex

7.   ____   characteristics, behaviours, and skills that are defined within a culture as being either masculine or feminine

8.   ____   surgery in which the person's genitals are changed to match his or her gender identity

9.   ____   a category of rapist whose actions are intended to degrade and humiliate the victim

10. ____ being genetically male but lacking a hormone responsible for shaping the penis and scrotum, resulting in ambiguous external genitalia

11. ____ a paraphilia characterised by recurrent, intense sexual urges involving touching and rubbing against a nonconsenting person

12. ____ a paraphilia in which a person becomes sexually aroused by observing unsuspecting people while they are undressing or involved in sexual activity

13. ____ a category of rapist with distorted views of sexuality and women, feelings of inferiority, and poor social skills

14. ____ a treatment where the therapist repeatedly presents the stimulus that elicits inappropriate sexual arousal in association with an aversive stimulus

15. ____ acts involving nonconsensual sexual penetration obtained by physical force, threat of bodily harm, or when the victim is incapable of giving consent

16. ____ a mental picture representing a person's ideal sexual relationship

17. ____ laws designed to keep some criminals in custody indefinitely

18. ____ a category of rapist with impulsive, unplanned actions who seeks immediate gratification

19. ____ laws which require the distribution of information to the public regarding the presence of child molesters and sexually violent offenders when they are released from prison

Names You Should Know — Matching

The following people have played an important role in research and theory of sexual and gender identity disorders. To test your knowledge, match the following names with the descriptions of their contributions to the study of abnormal psychology. Answers are listed at the end of the chapter.

a. Alfred Kinsey   c. Kurt Freund
b. William Masters and Virginia Johnson   d. John Money

1. ____ proposed a model of the human sexual response cycle and developed treatments for sexual dysfunctions

2. ____ applied scientific methods to the study of sexuality

3. ____ studied the etiology of paraphilias; developed the concept of lovemaps

4. ____ developed penile plethysmography, a method used to measure male sexual arousal and erotic preferences

Review of Concepts — Fill in the Blank and True/False

This section will help focus your studying by testing whether you understand the concepts presented in the text. After you have read and reviewed the material, test your comprehension and memory by filling in the following blanks or circling the right answer. Answers are listed at the end of the chapter.

1. Male and female orgasm have different numbers of stages: **true**   **false**

2. Women typically have a longer refractory period than men: **true**   **false**

3. Women are capable of multiple orgasms while men are typically not: **true**   **false**

4. Sexual problems are best seen as problems of the individual: **true**   **false**

5. Early scientific approaches to sexual behaviour were strongly influenced by the idea that the exclusive goal of sexuality was _____.

6. Kinsey rejected the distinction between _____ and _____ sexual behaviour and saw differences as quantitative rather than qualitative.

7. Men report that their sexual partners have orgasms more often than women report having orgasms: **true**   **false**

8. The only factor important to sexual satisfaction, especially among women, is experiencing an orgasm: **true**   **false**

9. Failure to reach orgasm is not considered a disorder unless it is _____ and results in _____.

10. Viagra has been documented to be effective in the treatment of erectile dysfunction: **true**   **false**

11. Viagra has been associated with some deaths: **true**   **false**

12. Hypoactive Sexual Desire Disorder can be diagnosed by comparing a person's interest level with a chart of normal levels of sexual interest: **true**   **false**

13. People with low sexual desire often have _____ disorders.

14. There are high correlations between subjective and physiological measures of arousal in normal women: **true**   **false**

15. Almost all clinicians will identify the response of ejaculating before or upon _____ or after _____ thrusts as premature ejaculation.

16. Dyspareunia is more common in   **men**   or   **women.**

17. What is the most frequent form of male sexual dysfunction?_____

18. There is a cultural prejudice against sexual activity among older_____.

19. Older men achieve erections **more quickly** or **more slowly**.

20. The subjective experience of the intensity of orgasm **increases** or **decreases** with age.

21. Frequency of sexual dysfunction among men typically **increases** or **decreases** with age.

22. Frequency of sexual dysfunction among women typically **increases** or **decreases** with age.

23. The influence of male sex hormones on sexual behaviour is thought to be on sexual _____ rather than on sexual _____.

24. Men who smoke cigarettes are more likely to have problems with _____.

25. Antidepressants can include the side-effect of orgasm problems: **true** **false**

26. Women born in more recent decades are less likely to be orgasmic: **true** **false**

27. Changing the way people think about sex is a major aspect of sex therapy:
    true **false**

28. Paraphilias are only diagnosed if the person has _____ the urges or is _____ by them.

29. Most of the people in treatment for sexual disorders are people with paraphilias:
    true **false**

30. The central feature of paraphilia is that sexual arousal is dependent on images that are detached from _____ relationships with another adult.

31. Paraphilias are similar to the _____.

32. Masochists tend to be disproportionately represented among poorer groups of people: **true** **false**

33. Paraphilia is most likely more common than what is estimated by community surveys: **true** **false**

34. A voyeur is not aroused by watching people who know they are being observed:
    true **false**

35. Most pedophiles are homosexual: **true   false**

36. Rape is not included as a paraphilia because it is not always motivated by

    _____.

37. Many rapists in one study had a history of paraphilias: **true   false**

38. Most people with a paraphilia exhibit other paraphilias as well: **true   false**

39. About what percent of people with paraphilias are men?   **60%   75%   95%**

40. Damage to what part of the brain can lead to unusual sexual behaviours?

    _____

41. _____ skills may play as important a role in paraphilias as sexual

    arousal.

42. A surprising number of people involved in masochism had what type of experience

    as children? _____

43. Most people in treatment for paraphilias are there _____.

44. Cognitive-behavioural treatment was found to be   **more**   or   **less**   effective

    than aversion therapy in treating paraphilia.

45. Gender identity disorders are relatively   **rare**   or   **common**.

46. Pseudohermaphrodites typically make a quick and fairly easy transition from a

    childhood female to an adult male gender identity: **true   false**

47. Results of sex-reassignment surgery have mostly been negative: **true   false**

Multiple Choice Questions

The following multiple choice questions will test your comprehension of the material presented in the chapter. Answers are listed at the end of the chapter.

1) All of the following types of medication have been used to treat paraphilias
   EXCEPT:

   a. antipsychotic medications   c. antianxiety medications
   b. antidepressants   d. all of the above have been used

2) According to Freund and Blanchard, all of the following factors may increase the probability that a person might experiment with unusual types of sexual stimulation or employ maladaptive sexual behaviours EXCEPT:

a. ignorance and poor understanding of human sexuality
b. lack of diverse sexual experiences
c. lack of self-esteem
d. lack of confidence and ability in social interactions

3) With regard to the context of occurrence, which of the following terms indicates that the sexual dysfunction is not limited only to certain situations or partners:

a. situational
b. lifelong
c. acquired
d. generalised

4) Recent revisions of the DSM reflect the following important changes in society's attitudes toward sexual behaviour EXCEPT:

a. growing acceptance of women of their own sexuality
b. tolerance for greater variety in human sexuality
c. society's complete acceptance of organized groups that represent specific forms of sexual orientation and expression
d. increased recognition that the main purpose of sexual behaviour need not be reproduction

5) _____ disorders are more common among women while _____ disorders are more common among men.

a. Orgasm; arousal
b. Arousal; orgasm
c. Aversion; desire
d. Desire; aversion

6. Studies show that most women seeking treatment for hypoactive sexual desire report all of the following EXCEPT:

a. negative perceptions of their parents' attitudes regarding sexual behaviour
b. a history of physical and sexual abuse
c. negative perceptions of their parents' demonstration of affection
d. feeling less close to their husbands and having fewer romantic feelings

7) This involves the use of nonliving objects for the purpose of sexual arousal.

a. frotteurism
b. pedophilia
c. fetishism
d. sexual masochism

8) Sex-reassignment surgery is the process whereby a person's genitals are changed to match his or her:

a. gender identity
b. sex role
c. sexual identity
d. gender role

9) According to your text, _____ may be the most common neurologically-based cause of impaired erectile responsiveness among men.

a. depression
b. coronary heart disease
c. diabetes
d. cancer

10) All of the following are treatment options for sexual dysfunctions EXCEPT:

a. sensate focus
b. cognitive restructuring
c. communication training
d. aversion therapy

11) _____ of the people who seek treatment for paraphilia disorders are men.

a. 40 percent
b. 60 percent
c. 75 percent
d. 95 percent

12) Gender Identity disorder appears to be strongly related to and may share a common aetiology with

a. transvestic fetishism
b. schizophrenia
c. pedophilia
d. sexual masochism

13) The sense of ourselves as being either male or female is known as:

a. sexual identity
b. gender dysphoria
c. gender identity
d. sex roles

14) Premature ejaculation may be the most frequent form of sexual dysfunction, affecting nearly 1 in every:

a. 5 adult men
b. 10 adult men
c.
d. 20 adult men

15) The treatment approach used for paraphilias in which the therapist repeatedly presents a stimulus eliciting inappropriate sexual arousal in association with an aversive stimulus is called:

a. counterconditioning
b. aversion therapy
c. flooding
d. systematic desensitisation

16) Research on sexual behaviour across the life span shows that:

a. younger men have difficulty regaining an erection if it is lost before orgasm, while older men can only maintain erections for a short period of time
b. older adults are not as interested in, or capable of, performing sexual behaviours as younger adults
c. differences between younger and older people are mostly a matter of degree
d. as women get older, the clitoris becomes more responsive

17) Men with this problem may report feeling aroused, but the vascular reflex mechanism fails, and sufficient blood is not pumped to the penis.

a. sexual aversion disorder
b. premature ejaculation
c. male orgasmic disorder
d. erectile dysfunction

18) In order to meet diagnostic criteria, all categories of sexual dysfunction require all of the following EXCEPT:

a. the sexual dysfunction is associated with atypical stimuli and the person is pre-occupied with, or consumed by, these activities
b. the disturbance causes marked distress or interpersonal difficulty
c. the sexual dysfunction is not better accounted for by another Axis I disorder (such as major depression)
d. the sexual dysfunction is not due to direct physiological effects of a substance or a general medical condition

19) Perhaps as many as _____ of females seeking treatment for hypoactive sexual desire report other forms of sexual dysfunction.

a. 25 percent
b. 40 percent
c. 60 percent
d. 75 percent

20) According to your text, sexual desire remains a controversial topic because:

a. it is so difficult to define
b. there is very little empirical research on sexual desire
c. it is a different construct for men than it is for women
d. all of the above

21) The unresponsiveness of most men to further engage in sexual stimulation for a period of time after reaching orgasm is called:

a. sensation of suspension
b. pulsation
c. sexual aversion
d. refractory period

22) Premature ejaculation might be present if a man is unable to delay ejaculation until his partner reaches orgasm at least _____ of the time.

a. 25 percent
b. 50 percent
c. 75 percent
d. 100 percent

23) Studies have shown that all of the following are important factors contributing to failure to reach orgasm among anorgasmic women EXCEPT:

a. failure to engage in effective behaviours during foreplay
b. negative attitudes toward masturbation
c. feelings of guilt about sex
d. failure to communicate effectively with their partner about sexual activities involving direct stimulation of the clitoris

24) All of the following refer to a sense of discomfort with one's anatomical sex EXCEPT:

    a. gender identity disorder   c. gender dysphoria
    b. transvestic fetishism   d. transsexualism

25) Research suggests that _____ of men over age 75 report experiencing erectile dysfunction.

    a. 30 percent   c. 50 percent
    b. 40 percent   d. 60 percent

26) This involves the act of observing an unsuspecting person who is naked, in the process of disrobing, or engaging in sexual activity:

    a. sexual sadism   c. exhibitionism
    b. voyeurism   d. fetishism

27) Which of the following characterises an individual who is genetically male, but is unable to produce a hormone that is responsible for shaping the penis and scrotum in the fetus, and is therefore born with external genitalia that are ambiguous in appearance?

    a. transsexualism
    b. secondary sexual characteristic disorder
    c. transvestic fetishism
    d. pseudohermaphroditism

28. Which of the following is NOT one of the reasons for opposition to the proposed diagnostic category of excessive sexual drive?

    a. it is very rare
    b. its definition is circular
    c. problems controlling sexual impulses can be characteristic of several other disorders
    d. it is unclear whether it represents a meaningful diagnostic category

Understanding Research — Fill in the Blank

Sexual Activity in the General Population: The text presents a detailed description of a study by Michael, Laumann, and Gagnon in the Research Close-Up. Finding the answers to these questions will help you get a good understanding of this study and why it is important. It is not necessary to memorize the answers; the process of finding them in the textbook will help you learn the material you need to know.

1. This study was the first large-scale followup to the _____ reports. How many men and women participated? _____ What ages were the subjects? _____ to _____. What was the most important element of the research design? The study used _____. During the year of the survey, _____ percent of the participants had more than one sexual partner, and _____ percent had no partner. What percent of people born between 1963 and 1974 have had premarital sex? _____ percent of men and _____ percent of women.

2. People without _____ affiliation felt less guilty about masturbating. Which was more prevalent, masturbation or anal sex? _____ Younger, better-educated people were more likely to use _____. When were people most reluctant to use condoms? _____

Hypothetical Constructs and Construct Validity: The text discusses these research issues in the Research Methods section. Finding the answers to these questions will help you get a good understanding of these issues.

3. Why is sexual arousal a hypothetical construct? _____

_____

Why is an erect penis not the same as sexual arousal? _____

_____

Sexual arousal is _____than the sum of feelings and responses that can be measured directly.

4. The penile plethysmograph records changes in penile _____.The vaginal photometer is probably most useful in measuring _____ to _____ levels of sexual arousal. These research devices are merely reflections of the construct of sexual arousal that has many _____.

Brief Essay

As a final exercise, write out answers to the following brief essay questions. Then compare your answers with the material presented in the text.

After you have answered these questions, review the "critical thinking" questions that are presented at the end of the text chapter. Answering these questions will help you integrate important issues and themes that have been featured throughout the chapter.

1.	Compare and contrast the treatment of paraphilias with the treatment of sexual dysfunction. Choose two types of paraphilias and two types of sexual dysfunctions and discuss which type of treatment would be most effective for each of them.

2.	Discuss David Barlow's series of studies comparing sexually dysfunctional men with control subjects in laboratory settings. What were his findings? What are some of the possible limitations to these studies? What are the applications of his findings?

3.	Compare and contrast the different proposals regarding the etiology of paraphilias as presented in your text. Which proposal(s) do you believe best explains the aetiology of paraphilias? Why?

ANSWER KEY

Key Terms — Matching #1

1. f	8. j	15. q
2. d	9. b	16. n
3. l	10. o	17. r
4. p	11. c	18. m
5. i	12. g	19. h
6. a	13. k	
7. s	14. e	

Names You Should Know

1. b
2. a
3. d
4. c

Key Terms — Matching #2

a. 3	k. 6	
b. 1	l. 2	
c. 9	m. 13	
d. 15	n. 7	
e. 19	o. 17	
f. 18	p. 5	
g. 8	q. 14	
h. 12	r. 10	
i. 11	s. 16	
j. 20	t. 4	

Key Terms — Matching #3

1. a	11. c
2. g	12. b
3. e	13. i
4. h	14. m
5. d	15. f
6. q	16. l
7. p	17. o
8. s	18. k
9. j	19. n
10. r	

Multiple Choice

1. a	6. b	11. d	16. c	21. d	26. b
2. b	7. c	12. a	17. d	22. b	27. d
3. d	8. a	13. c	18. a	23. a	28. a
4. c	9. c	14. a	19. d	24. b	
5. a	10. d	15. b	20. a	25. c	

Review of Concepts

1. true
2. false
3. true
4. false
5. reproduction
6. normal and abnormal
7. true
8. false
9. persistent; distress
10. true
11. true
12. false
13. mood
14. false
15. insertion
16. women
17. premature ejaculation
18. women
19. more slowly
20. decreases
21. increases
22. decreases
23. appetite; performance
24. erection
25. true
26. false
27. true
28. acted on; distressed
29. false
30. loving
31. addictions
32. false
33. true
34. true
35. false
36. sexual arousal
37. true
38. true
39. 95 percent
40. temporal lobe
41. Interpersonal
42. traumatic disease and painful medical procedures
43. involuntarily
44. more
45. rare
46. true
47. false

Understanding Research

1. Kinsey; 3,500; 18 to 59; probability sampling; 16 percent; 11 percent; 84 percent; 80 percent

2. religious; masturbation; condoms; in new sexual relationships

3. because it cannot be observed directly; it is not always accompanied by subjective arousal; more

4. tumescence; moderate; low; dimensions

CHAPTER 13
SCHIZOPHRENIC DISORDERS

Chapter Outline

C. Psychological Factors
   1. Family Interaction
   2. Expressed Emotion
D. Integration and Multiple Pathways
E. The Search for Markers of Vulnerability
   1. Attention and Cognition
   2. Eye-Tracking Dysfunction

VI. Treatment
  A. Antipsychotic Medication
    1. Side Effects
    2. Maintenance Medication
    3. Atypical Antipsychotics
  B. Psychosocial Treatment
    1. Family-Oriented Aftercare
    2. Social Skills Training
    3. Cognitive-Behavioural Therapy
    4. Assertive Community Treatment
    5. Institutional Programs

Learning Objectives

After reviewing the material presented in this chapter, you should be able to:

1. Distinguish between positive symptoms, negative symptoms, and disorganization.

2. Distinguish the prodromal, active, and residual phases of schizophrenia.

3. Define and describe hallucinations, delusional beliefs, and disorganised speech.

4. Provide examples of typical motor disturbances, affective and emotional disturbances, and avolition.

5. Know the contributions of Kraepelin and Bleuler in defining schizophrenia.

6. Distinguish disorganised, catatonic, paranoid, undifferentiated, and residual types of schizophrenia using DSM-IV criteria.

7. Describe the following related disorders: schizoaffective disorders, delusional disorder, brief psychotic disorders.

8. Know the basic epidemiological statistics for incidence and prevalence of the disorder, as well as gender differences in age of onset.

9. Understand the genetic evidence for schizophrenia, which leads to a diathesis-stres model of aetiology.

10. Describe some of the research that has discovered structural brain abnormalities for schizophrenics.

11. Explain the dopamine hypothesis and current beliefs about the role of dopamine in schizophrenia.

12. Identify some social and psychological factors that may contribute to the development and/or maintenance of schizophrenia.

13. Understand the significance of research that has identified attentional, cognitive, and eye-tracking dysfunctions in schizophrenics and their biological relatives.

14. Describe the effectiveness of neuroleptic medication and atypical antipsychotic medications and the relevant side effects that are involved in such treatments.

15. Provide a description of family-oriented aftercare programs, social skills training, cognitive-behaviour therapy, and institutional programs in which token economy systems may be used.

Key Terms — Matching #1

The following terms related to schizophrenia are important to know. To test your knowledge, match the following terms with their definitions. Answers are listed at the end of the chapter.

a   Negative symptoms
b.   Positive symptoms
c.   Disorganization
d.   Schizophreniform disorder
e.   Active phase
f.   Prodromal phase
g.   Residual phase
h.   Hallucinations
i.   Disorganised speech
j.   Stuporous state
k.   Incoherent
l.   Loose associations
m.   Tangentiality

n.   Perseveration
o.   Alogia
p.   Poverty of speech
q.   Thought blocking
r.   Catatonia
s.   Delusions
t.   Blunted affect
u.   Anhedonia
v.   Inappropriate affect
w.   Avolition
x.   Dementia praecox
y.   Catatonic type
z.   Disorganised type

1. ____ the patient's train of speech is interrupted before a thought is completed
2. ____ when hallucinations, delusions, and disorganised speech are evident
3. ____ after positive symptoms; continued deterioration of role functioning
4. ____ reflect loss of normal functions
5. ____ immobility and marked muscular rigidity, or excitement and overactivity
6. ____ extremely disorganised speech which conveys little meaning

7. _____ an early grouping of several types of psychosis now seen as schizophrenia
8. _____ reflect a distortion of normal functions, like psychosis
9. _____ inability to experience pleasure
10. _____ remarkable reductions in the amount of speech
11. _____ schizophrenia characterised by disorganised speech, disorganised behaviour, and flat or inappropriate affect
12. _____ shifting topics too abruptly
13. _____ schizophrenia characterised by symptoms of motor immobility or excessive and purposeless motor activity
14. _____ psychotic symptoms lasting between 1 and 6 months
15. _____ idiosyncratic beliefs that are rigidly held despite their preposterous nature
16. _____ indecisiveness, ambivalence, and loss of willpower
17. _____ generally reduced responsiveness
18. _____ persistently repeating the same word or phrase over and over again
19. _____ prior to positive symptoms, marked by deterioration in role functioning
20. _____ a flattening or restriction of a person's nonverbal display of emotion
21. _____ incongruity and lack of adaptability in emotional expression
22. _____ severe disruptions of verbal communication involving the form of speech
23. _____ replying to a question with an irrelevant response
24. _____ impoverished thinking marked by nonfluent or barren speech
25. _____ verbal communication problems and bizarre behaviour
26. _____ sensory experiences not caused by actual external stimuli

Key Terms — Matching #2

The following terms related to schizophrenia are important to know. To test your knowledge, match the following terms with their definitions. Answers are listed at the end of the chapter.

1. Paranoid type
2. Undifferentiated type
3. Residual type
4. Schizoaffective disorder
5. Delusional disorder
6. Brief psychotic disorder
7. Phenothiazines
8. Lateral ventricles
9. Magnetic resonance imaging
10. Hemispheric asymmetry
11. Treatment resistance
12. Assertive community treatment
13. Positron emission tomography

14. Dopamine hypothesis
15. Social causation hypothesis
16. Social selection hypothesis
17. Communication deviance
18. Expressed emotion
19. Case control design
20. Schizotaxia
21. Threshold model
22. Vulnerability marker
23. Neuroleptic drugs
24. Extrapyramidal symptoms
25. Tardive dyskinesia
26. Atypical antipsychotics

a. _____ harmful events associated with membership in lowest social classes play a causal role in the development of schizophrenia

b. _____ subtle neurological defect in people predisposed to schizophrenia

c. _____ an imaging technique that allows identification of specific, small brain structures

d. _____ comparisons between groups of people with a disorder and groups of people who do not have the disorder

e. _____ side effects including muscular rigidity, tremors, restless agitation, peculiar involuntary postures, and motor inertia

f. _____ the cavities on each side of the brain that are filled with cerebrospinal fluid

g. _____ an imaging technique that reflects changes in brain activity as the person performs various tasks

h. _____ focuses on the function of specific dopamine pathways in the limbic area of the brain as having a role in the aetiology of schizophrenia

i. _____ schizophrenia characterised by psychotic symptoms but that does not fit any one subtype

j. _____ antipsychotic medications that induce side effects that resemble the motor symptoms of Parkinson's disease

k. _____ an intervention combining psychological treatments with medication

l. _____ schizophrenia characterised by systematic delusions with persecutory or grandiose content

m. _____ a specific measure that might be useful in identifying people who are vulnerable to a disorder

n. _____ an episode of symptoms of both schizophrenia and a mood disorder

o. _____ people with schizophrenia experience downward social mobility

p. _____ peculiar statements, difficulty in completing answers, and other types of disruptive verbal behaviour in parents of schizophrenics

q. _____ does not meet the criteria of schizophrenia but are preoccupied for at least one month with delusions that are not bizarre

r. _____ the first antipsychotic medication to be used in North America

s. _____ negative or intrusive attitudes displayed by relatives of schizophrenics

t. _____ a syndrome caused by prolonged treatment with neuroleptic drugs consisting of involuntary movements of the mouth and face as well as spasmodic movements of the limbs and trunk of the body

u. _____ people who exhibit psychotic symptoms for at least a day but less than a month

v. _____ new forms of antipsychotic medication that do not produce extrapyramidal symptoms or tardive dyskinesia

w. _____ a structure being larger in one hemisphere of the brain than the other

x. _____ liability to have a disorder lies along a continuum, but the probability that certain symptoms will be present changes dramatically as the person crosses a certain point on the continuum

y. _____ failure to improve on three types of medication after six weeks of treatment

z. _____ schizophrenia in partial remission, with no active phase symptoms

Names You Should Know — Matching

The following people have played an important role in research and theory of schizophrenic disorders. To test your knowledge, match the following names with the descriptions of their contributions to the study of abnormal psychology. Answers are listed at the end of the chapter.

a. Emil Kraeplin

b. Eugen Bleuler

c. Lyman Wynne & Margaret Singer

d. Kurt Schneider

e. Irving Gottesman

f. Leonard Heston

g. Paul Meehl

h. Heinz Lehmann

1. ____ one of the world's leading experts on genetic factors and schizophrenia
2. ____ grouped together several psychotic disorders into the category of dementia praecox, an early term for schizophrenia
3. ____ proposed a theory of schizophrenia involving schizotaxia
4. ____ conducted the first adoption study of schizophrenia
5. ____ developed a diagnostic system for schizophrenia which emphasised first-rank symptoms
6. ____ coined the term schizophrenia, which means splitting of mental associations
7. ____ the first North American physician use chlorpromazine to treat schizophrenia
8. ____ explored communication deviance among parents of schizophrenics

Review of Concepts — Fill in the Blank and True/False

This section will help focus your studying by testing whether you understand the concepts presented in the text. After you have read and reviewed the material, test your comprehension and memory by filling in the following blanks or circling the right answer. Answers are listed at the end of the chapter.

1. What are the three categories of symptoms of schizophrenia? _____ _____ and _____

2. What is the period of risk for the development of a first episode of schizophrenia? _____ years old to _____ years old

3. After the onset of schizophrenia, most people return to their previous levels of functioning: **true**   **false**

4. What is the most common type of hallucination? _____

5. Delusions are typically shared by the patient's family: **true**   **false**

6. Disorganised speech breaks all the rules of grammar: **true**   **false**

7. During a stuporous state, schizophrenic patients remain aware of what is happening around them: **true   false**

8. Many people with schizophrenia evidence social withdrawal: **true   false**

9. Schizophrenia is a sort of multiple personality disorder: **true   false**

10. Schizophrenia follows a predictable course among most patients: **true   false**

11. What is the lifetime morbid risk of schizophrenia? _____ percent

12. Women typically have an earlier age of onset than men: **true   false**

13. Men typically have more negative symptoms than women: **true   false**

14. Women typically respond better to treatment than men: **true   false**

15. Schizophrenia is very rare in developing countries: **true   false**

16. People with schizophrenia have a better outcome if they live in a developing country rather than a developed country: **true   false**

17. What is the lifetime risk of developing schizophrenia if your identical twin has the disorder? _____ percent

18. What is the lifetime risk of developing schizophrenia if your fraternal twin has the disorder? _____ percent

19. Genetic factors do not play a role in the aetiology of schizophrenia:
     true   false

20. Adoption studies indicate that environmental factors cause schizophrenia:
     true   false

21. The data suggest that multiple genes are responsible for vulnerability to schizophrenia: **true   false**

22. The lifetime prevalence of schizophrenia is: _____

23. Male schizophrenics experience more _____ symptoms relative to female schizophrenics.

24. Linkage studies indicate that _____ of people with a small deletion on chromosome _____ develop schizophrenia.

25. People with schizophrenia have been found to have _____ lateral ventricles in the brain.

26. People with schizophrenia are more likely to show a decrease in the size of what brain structure? _____

27. One MZ twin pair discordant for schizophrenia involved one brother who was a successful businessman and another who was severely impaired with schizophrenia. Whose lateral ventricles were five times larger?

    _____

28. What other neurotransmitter besides dopamine may be involved in schizophrenia?

    _____

29. Which hypothesis has received support in the research literature, the social causation hypothesis or the social selection hypothesis? _____

30. Parents of schizophrenic children who show communication deviance in their conversations with their ill children **do** or **do not** show CD in their conversations with their well children.

31. Men with schizophrenia were **more** or **less** likely to return to the hospital if they were discharged to live with their wives or parents rather than their siblings or strangers.

32. What seems to be the important component of expressed emotion?_____

33. Lots of contact with relatives high on EE **helps** or **hurts** patients with schizophrenia; and lots of contact with relatives low on EE **helps** or **hurts** patients with schizophrenia.

34. High EE is **more** or **less** common in Western countries.

35. Schizophrenic patients are **more** or **less** accurate than normal people in the Continuous Performance Task.

36. Relatives of schizophrenic patients are **more** or **less** accurate than normal people in the Continuous Performance Task.

37. _____-tracking performance may be associated with a predisposition to schizophrenia.

38. Neuroleptic medications take _____ to have an effect.

39. All people with schizophrenia respond to neuroleptic medications given in the correct dose: **true**   **false**

40. What percent of patients develop tardive dyskinesia after long-term treatment with neuroleptic drugs? _____ percent

41. Continued maintenance on neuroleptic drugs after recovery significantly reduces relapse: **true**   **false**

42. Why is Clozaril not used with all schizophrenic patients? _____

_____

43. Patients who do not respond to neuroleptic medication do not improve with any type of treatment: **true**   **false**

44. Cognitive-behavioural therapy for schizophrenia has been shown to be effective at reducing the symptoms of schizophrenia: **true**   **false**

Multiple Choice Questions

The following multiple choice questions will test your comprehension of the material presented in the chapter. Answers are listed at the end of the chapter.

1) Research on the relationship between expressed emotion (EE) and schizophrenia supports which of the following?

   a. the presence of expressed emotion is only associated with the onset of an individual's initial episode of schizophrenia
   b. among the various types of comments that contribute to a high EE rating, criticism is typically most associated with the likelihood of relapse
   c. the influence of expressed emotions is unique to schizophrenia
   d. all of the above

2) The trend in the DSM diagnosis of schizophrenia over time has been which of the following?

   a. include more affective symptoms
   b. omit subtyping of the disorder
   c. move from a broader to narrower definition of schizophrenia
   d. move from a more restrictive to less restrictive duration criterion

3) Which of the following would NOT be considered a positive symptom of schizophrenia?

    a. hallucinations   c. delusions
    b. blunted affect   d. disorganised speech

4) The distribution of schizophrenia within families is probably best explained by which of the following genetic models?

    a. polygenic   c. single recessive gene
    b. single dominant gene   d. linked genes

5) A difference between schizophrenia and delusional disorder is that:

    a. patients with schizophrenia display less impairment in their daily functioning than patients with delusional disorder
    b. patients with delusional disorder display more negative symptoms during the active phase of their illness
    c. the behaviour of patients with schizophrenia is considerably less bizarre
    d. patients with delusional disorder are preoccupied with delusions that are not necessarily considered bizarre

6) In the search to identify people who are vulnerable to schizophrenia, several potential vulnerability markers have been considered. Which of the following would NOT be considered a good criterion for a vulnerability marker?

    a. the marker should be able to distinguish between people who are already schizophrenic and people who are not
    b. the marker should be a characteristic which is stable over time
    c. the marker should be able to identify more people who are relatives of schizophrenics than people in the general population
    d. the marker should be able to predict the likelihood of relapse for people who have already experienced their first episode of schizophrenia

7) Individuals who exhibit psychotic symptoms for no more than a month and that cannot be attributed to other disorders such as substance abuse or mood disorder usually receive the diagnosis of:

    a. delusional disorder   c. brief psychotic disorder
    b. schizophreniform disorder   d. schizoaffective disorder

8) Tangentiality is an example of which type of disturbance?

    a. motor disturbance   c. disorganised speech
    b. affective disturbance   d. delusional belief

9) Which of the following statements is TRUE regarding the use of neuroleptic medication?

   a. beneficial effects are noticed within 24 hours after beginning the medication
   b. they appear to be particularly effective for relief of the positive symptoms associated with schizophrenia
   c. almost all schizophrenic patients are considered to be complete responders to this type of medication
   d. schizophrenic patients with the most severe symptoms respond best to them

10) Research on schizophrenic twins and adopted-away offspring of schizophrenics suggests which of the following?

    a. vulnerability to schizophrenia is consistently manifested by the same symptoms of this disorder across relatives
    b. vulnerability to schizophrenia is expressed through a variety of different symptom patterns, including depressive and anxiety syndromes
    c. vulnerability to schizophrenia is consistently manifested by the same symptoms of this disorder only when male relatives are affected
    d. vulnerability to schizophrenia is sometimes manifested by schizophrenialike personality traits and non-schizophrenic psychotic disorders

11) Which of the following is NOT a possible explanation for the relationship between the presence of familial communication problems and schizophrenia?

    a. parental communication problems may cause the child's disorder
    b. the child's adjustment problems may cause the parents' problems
    c. both the child's disorder and the parent communication problems reflect a common genetic influence
    d. all of the above are possible explanations for the presence of this relationship

12) Which of the following reflects a change in the DSM-IV definition of schizophrenia?

    a. negative symptoms assume a more prominent role
    b. positive symptoms assume a more prominent role
    c. the person must display active symptoms of the illness for at least one year
    d. a decline in the person's functioning is no longer required

13) A restriction of an individual's nonverbal display of his or her emotional responses is referred to as:

    a. blunted affect   c. anhedonia
    b. affective loosening   d. inappropriate affect

14) An interesting and consistent result across numerous MRI studies is that some people with schizophrenia have:

    a. an enlarged hypothalamus   c. enlarged temporal lobes
    b. enlarged lateral ventricles   d. less cerebrospinal fluid

15) Studies investigating the relationship between social class and schizophrenia support that risk for the disorder:

   a. is associated with adverse social and economic circumstances
   b. is not associated by circumstances most likely to be present in the lives of people who are economically disadvantaged
   c. is associated with the unique types of circumstances most frequently affiliated with high social class
   d. is most associated with recent immigration to a country

16) Which statement about the course of schizophrenia is TRUE?

   a. a significant amount of individuals experience their first episode between 35-50 years of age
   b. the onset of the disorder typically occurs during adolescence or early adulthood
   c. the active phase of illness is always the longest of the three phases
   d. the premorbid phase of illness usually lasts no longer than six months

17) Inconsistencies associated with the dopamine model of schizophrenia include which of the following?

   a. dopamine blockage begins immediately when medication is administered but the drugs often take several days to become effective
   b. some patients do not respond positively to drugs that block dopamine receptors
   c. studies investigating the byproducts of dopamine in cerebrospinal fluid are inconsisent and inconclusive
   d. all of the above

18) Which of the following is NOT included in the DSM-IV as a subtype of schizophrenia?

   a. paranoid   c. undifferentiated
   b. residual   d. negative

19) Joshua's behaviour has been observed on the hospital ward for several hours. He has been sitting perfectly still in one position. Furthermore, he has been completely mute (has not spoken a single word) since admission. Which subtype of schizophrenia best represents Joshua's behaviour?

   a. disorganised   c. catatonic
   b. paranoid   d. undifferentiated

20) The Danish high-risk for schizophrenia project has supported which of the following hypotheses?

   a. families with individuals who develop the positive symptoms of the disorder appear to be at higher genetic risk
   b. children who experience head injuries before age five appear to be at greater risk for schizophrenia

c. neurodevelopmental problems in schizophrenia are antecedents rather than consequences of the disorder

d. problems in delivery at birth do not appear to be associated with vulnerability to schizophrenia

21) A criticism of twin studies and their persuasive evidence for the role of genetic factors in schizophrenia is that:

a. DZ and MZ twin concordance rates are approximately equal, suggesting that genetic factors are less important than environmental factors

b. MZ twins, because of their physical similarity, are probably treated more similarly by their parents than even DZ twins, which confounds environmental with genetic factors

c. the studies determining concordance rates are flawed because they do not take into account the birth order of the MZ twins

d. the concordance rates for MZ twins for schizophrenia has fluctuated dramatically across studies

22) The potentially exciting part of eye-tracking dysfunction and the possibility of this characteristic being a vulnerability marker for schizophrenia is that:

a. eye-tracking dysfunction appears to be influenced by genetic factors and is apparently a stable trait

b. eye-tracking dysfunction appears to be present only in patients with schizophrenia

c. approximately 90 percent of the first-degree relatives of schizophrenic individuals show this characteristic

d. the eye-tracking dysfunction only appears during episodes of schizophrenia

23) Research suggests that the outcome of schizophrenia may be best described by which of the following statements?

a. 50 percent of the individuals continue to deteriorate after their first episode, 10 percent completely recover, and 40 percent experience intermittent episodes

b. 30 percent of the individual recover fairly well after their initial episode, 30 percent continue to deteriorate, and 40 percent continue to experience intermittent episodes

c. approximately 60 percent of the individuals recover fairly well after their initial episode, while 40 percent continue to deteriorate

d. approximately 60 percent of the individuals continue to deteriorate after their initial episode, while 40 percent continue to experience intermittent episodes

24) When Samuel grins as he talks about the loss of his father in a traumatic accident, he is displaying:

a. disorganised affect

b. avolition

c. catatonia

d. inappropriate affect

25) The theory that harmful events associated with being a member of the lowest social class (e.g., poor nutrition, social isolation) play a role in the development of schizophrenia is called:

a. the social class hypothesis
b. the social causation hypothesis
c. the social impairment hypothesis
d. the social selection hypothesis

26) The usefulness of subtyping schizophrenia has been criticized because:

a. some individuals do not fit the traditional subtype descriptions
b. some individuals display the symptoms of more than one subtype simultaneously
c. the symptoms of some individuals change from one episode to the next, reflecting subtype instability
d. all of the above

27) The average concordance rate for monozygotic twins for schizophrenia is:

a. 22 percent
b. 36 percent
c. 48 percent
d. 72 percent

28) Perhaps the most unpleasant side effect of neuroleptics is:

a. the fact that the drugs must be taken for two to four months before the patient experiences relief from symptoms
b. potentially toxic reactions to the drugs if the patient's diet is not carefully monitored
c. the presence of extrapyramidal symptoms
d. acute gastrointestinal symptoms (e.g., nausea, vomiting) during the first few weeks of use

29) Research on gender differences in schizophrenia supports that:

a. men experience their first episode of schizophrenia about five years later than women
b. women typically display better premorbid social competence prior to their first episode of schizophrenia
c. men typically display a less chronic course compared to women
d. women display more negative symptoms

30) Bleuler's definition of schizophrenia emphasized which of the following?

a. signs and symptoms of the disorder
b. course and outcome
c. genetic vulnerability markers
d. impairment in social roles

Understanding Research — Fill in the Blank

The Danish High-Risk Project: The text presents a detailed description of a study by Mednick and Schulsinger in the Research Close-Up. Finding the answers to these questions will help you get a good understanding of this study and why it is important. It is not necessary to memorize the answers; the process of finding them in the textbook will help you learn the material you need to know.

1. What was the high-risk group used in this study? _____

    _____ What percent of the sample was expected to

    develop schizophrenia? _____ percent. How many subjects were there all

    together? _____ The children in the comparison group came from families

    that had been free of mental illness for at least _____ generations. Data came from

    _____ records at the time of birth, structured _____

    interviews, and _____ scans.

2. How many of the high-risk offspring have developed schizophrenia? _____
    What percent of the high-risk offspring have developed schizotypal personality

    disorder? _____ percent. Rates of mood disorders were _____ in the

    high-risk and the control groups. Delivery complications and enlarged ventricles

    were _____ in the high-risk but not the low-risk group. The members

    of the high-risk group who did develop schizophrenia had _____ pregnancy

    and birth complications than those who did not develop the disorder.

Comparison Groups in Psychopathology Research: The text discusses this research issue in the Research Methods section. Finding the answers to these questions will help you get a good understanding of these issues.

3. A case control design depends on comparisons between _____

    and _____. How much finding a difference between these

    groups indicates that difference is causally related to the disorder depends on

    whether the _____ was appropriate. What are two types of

    comparison groups? _____ and _____.

4. Lack of specificity of a particular variable to the particular disorder may suggest

    that the variable is not a cause of the disorder but a _____ of

    being mentally ill or being treated in a psychiatric hospital. Expressed emotion predicts relapse among schizophrenic patients and also among

_____. However, expressed

emotion is clearly still an _____ variable.

Brief Essay

As a final exercise, write out answers to the following brief essay questions. Then compare your answers with the material presented in the text.

   After you have answered these questions, review the "critical thinking" questions that are presented at the end of the text chapter. Answering these questions will help you integrate important issues and themes that have been featured throughout the chapter.

1.   Pretend that you are on the committee that will be responsible for developing the definition for schizophrenia (i.e., the diagnostic criteria) for DSM-V. Signs and symptoms, duration of episodes, degree of impairment, familial, biological, genetic data, etc.— what would you consider to be the most appropriate criteria to be included in your definition and why?

2.   Explain what is meant by the diathesis-stress model of schizophrenia. Which factors reviewed in your text would represent the diathesis? Which factors would represent stress?

3.   Review the questions and considerations that an investigator must address as she designs a research project in psychopathology, comparing patients with a certain diagnosis with a comparison group. What are the issues involved in the selection of a meaningful comparison group?

4.   Briefly describe and compare the three forms of psychosocial treatment reviewed in your textbook that have been shown to be effective for schizophrenia. What are their advantages and disadvantages as treatment programs?

ANSWER KEY

Key Terms — Matching #1

1. q	10. p	19. f
2. e	11. z	20. t
3. g	12. l	21. v
4. a	13. y	22. i
5. r	14. d	23. m
6. k	15. s	24. o
7. x	16. w	25. c
8. b	17. j	26. h
9. u	18. n	

Names You Should Know

1. e
2. a
3. g
4. f
5. d
6. b
7. h
8. c

Key Term — Matching #2

a. 15	g. 13	m. 22	s. 18	y. 11
b. 20	h. 14	n. 4	t. 25	z. 3
c. 9	i. 2	o. 16	u. 6	
d. 19	j. 23	p. 17	v. 26	
e. 24	k. 12	q. 5	w. 10	
f. 8	l. 1	r. 7	x. 21	

Multiple Choice

1. b	7. c	13. a	19. c	25. b
2. c	8. c	14. b	20. c	26. d
3. b	9. b	15. a	21. b	27. c
4. a	10. d	16. b	22. a	28. c
5. d	11. d	17. d	23. b	29. b
6. d	12. a	18. d	24. d	30. a

Review of Concepts

1. positive symptoms; negative symptoms; and disorganization
2. 20; 35
3. false
4. auditory
5. false
6. false
7. true
8. true
9. false
10. false
11. 1 percent
12. false
13. true
14. true
15. false
16. true
17. 48 percent
18. 17 percent
19. false
20. false
21. true
22. .5 to 1.5%
23. negative and chronic
24. 25%; 22
25. larger
26. left temporal lobe
27. the businessman
38. serotonin
29. both
30. do not
31. more
32. criticism
33. hurts; helps
34. more
35. less
36. less
37. Eye
38. several weeks
39. true
40. 20 percent
41. true
42. causes fatal agranulocytosis in 1 percent of patients
43. false
44. true

Understanding Research

1. children of schizophrenic patients; 13 percent; 311; three; hospital; diagnostic; CT

2. 31; 18 percent; similar; correlated; more

3. cases and a control group; comparison; normal participants and patient controls

4. consequence; patients with mood disorders; important

CHAPTER 14
DEMENTIA, DELIRIUM, AND AMNESTIC DISORDERS

Chapter Outline

I. Overview

II. Typical Symptoms and Associated Features
    A. Delirium
    B. Dementia
        1. Cognitive Symptoms
            a. Memory and Learning
            b. Verbal Communication
            c. Perception
            d. Abstract Thinking
            e. Judgement and Social Behaviour
        2. Assessment of Cognitive Impairment
        3. Associated Features
    C. Amnestic Disorder

III. Classification
    A. Brief Historical Perspective
    B. DSM-IV and DSM-IV-TR
    C. Specific Disorders
        1. Dementia of the Alzheimer's Type
        2. Pick's Disease
        3. Huntington's Disease
        4. Parkinson's Disease
        5. Vascular Dementia
        6. Dementia with Lewy Bodies
        7. Dementia versus Depression

IV. Epidemiology of Delirium and Dementia
    A. Prevalence of Dementia
    B. Prevalence by Subtypes of Dementia
    C. Cross-Cultural Comparisons

V. Aetiological Considerations and Research
    A. Delirium
    B. Dementia
        1. Genetic Factors
        2. Neurotransmitters
        3. Viral Infections
        4. Immune System Dysfunction
        5. Environmental Factors

VI. Treatment and Management
   A. Medication
   B. Environmental and Behavioural Management
   C. Support for Caregivers

Learning Objectives

After reviewing the material presented in this chapter, you should be able to:

1. Define and distinguish dementia, delirium, and amnestic disorders.

2. Provide the basic symptoms of delirium.

3. Distinguish retrograde from anterograde amnesia.

4. Describe the primary symptoms of aphasia, apraxia, and agnosia.

5. Identify the functions of neuropsychological assessment in diagnosis of dementia.

6. Describe some of the primary features of amnestic disorder and distinguish them from dementia.

7. Identify the key contributions of Pinel, Broca, Wernicke, Korsakoff, Alzheimer, and Kraepelin in the diagnosis of cognitive disorders.

8. Distinguish primary from secondary dementia—and differentiated from undifferentiated primary dementia.

9. Describe some of the features of Alzheimer's, Pick's, Huntington's, Parkinson's, and vascular diseases.

10. Describe the role of genetics, neurotransmitters, viral infections, and environmental factors in the development of cognitive disorders.

11. Know the importance of accurate diagnosis in the treatment of dementia.

12. Discuss the importance of environmental and behavioural management as well as caregiver support and respite programs in treatment of the patient suffering from a cognitive disorder.

Key Terms — Matching #1

The following terms related to dementia, delirium, and amnestic disorders are important to know. To test your knowledge, match the following terms with their definitions. Answers are listed at the end of the chapter.

a.	Dementia	j.	Aphasia
b.	Delirium	k.	Apraxia
c.	Amnestic disorders	l.	Agnosia
d.	Neurologists	m.	Neuropsychological assessment
e.	Neuropsychologists	n.	Dyskinesia
f.	Mechanics	o.	Korsakoff's syndrome
g.	Pragmatics	p.	Primary dementia
h.	Retrograde amnesia	q.	Secondary dementia
i.	Anterograde amnesia		

1. ____ a gradually worsening loss of memory and related cognitive functions
2. ____ inability to learn or remember new material after a particular point in time
3. ____ a disorder caused by chronic alcoholism characterised by memory impairment
4. ____ problems identifying stimuli in the environment
5. ____ cognitive impairment is produced by the direct effect of a disease on brain tissue
6. ____ a confusional state that develops over a short period of time and is often associated with agitation and hyperactivity
7. ____ involuntary movements such as tics and tremors
8. ____ fluid intelligence, the "hardware" of the mind
9. ____ psychologists with expertise in the assessment of specific types of cognitive impairment
10. ____ various types of loss or impairment in language caused by brain damage
11. ____ evaluation of performance on psychological tests to indicate whether a person has a brain disorder
12. ____ physicians who deal primarily with diseases of the brain and nervous system
13. ____ a cognitive disorder characterised by limited memory impairments
14. ____ difficulty performing purposeful movements in response to verbal commands
15. ____ cognitive impairment is a by-product or side effect of some other type of biological or psychological dysfunction
16. ____ loss of memory for events prior to the onset of an illness or traumatic event
17. ____ crystallised intelligence, the "software" of the mind

Key Terms — Matching #2

The following terms related to dementia, delirium, and amnestic disorders are important to know. To test your knowledge, match the following terms with their definitions. Answers are listed at the end of the chapter.

1. Alzheimer's disease
2. Tauproteins
3. Neurofibrillary tangles
4. Senile plaques

5. Beta-amyloid
6. Pick's disease
7. Pick's bodies
8. Huntington's disease

9. Chorea
10. Parkinson's disease
11. Infarct
12. Vascular dementia
13. Pseudodementia

14. Autosomal dominant trait
15. Genetic linkage
16. Creutzfeldt-Jakob disease
17. Respite programs
18. Lewy bodies

a. ____ a protein material
b. ____ caused by a dominant gene not located on one of the sex chromosomes
c. ____ a lesion consisting of a central core of homogenous protein material surrounded by clumps of debris left over from destroyed neurons
d. ____ a distinctive ballooning of nerve cells
e. ____ reinforce microtubules; lacking in patients with Alzheimer's Disease
f. ____ a form of dementia associated with atrophy in the frontal and temporal lobes of the brain
g. ____ a close association between to genes on a chromosome
h. ____ disorder of the motor system caused by a degeneration of the substantia nigra and loss of dopamine but rarely including dementia
i. ____ provide caregivers with temporary periods of relief from caring for a demented patient
j. ____ symptoms of dementia actually produced by a major depressive disorder
k. ____ a form of dementia characterised by the presence of unusual involuntary muscle movements as well as personality changes
l. ____ a form of dementia in which cognitive impairment appears gradually and deterioration is progressive
m. ____ a form of dementia produced by a slow-acting virus
n. ____ the area of dead tissue produced by a stroke
o. ____ a form of dementia associated with strokes
p. ____ when the structural network of some neurofibrils becomes highly disorganised
q. ____ unusual involuntary muscle movements
r. ____ deposits found in neurons of patients with Parkinson's disease and dementia

Review of Concepts — Fill in the Blank and True/False

This section will help focus your studying by testing whether you understand the concepts presented in the text. After you have read and reviewed the material, test your comprehension and memory by filling in the following blanks or circling the right answer. Answers are listed at the end of the chapter.

1. Delirium can fluctuate throughout the day: **true   false**

2. Delirium is less common among the elderly: **true   false**

3. Dementia can be cured: **true   false**

4. Changes in cognitive processes are not a normal part of aging: **true   false**

5. Which of the following typically show a decline with age: **mechanics   pragmatics**

6. Neuropsychological tests can sometimes be used to infer the location of a brain lesion: **true   false**

7. Hallucinations and delusions are seen in what percent of dementia cases: _____

8. Korsakoff's syndrome may be caused in part by a _____ deficiency.

9. Which types of dementia are most common: **differentiated   undifferentiated**

10. A definitive diagnosis of Alzheimer's disease can only be made after _____.

11. Huntington's disease is caused by _____.

12. Vascular dementia often results in **unilateral** or **bilateral** impairment.

13. Almost _____ percent of people over 65 years of age exhibit symptoms of moderate or severe dementia: **8   20   60**

14. Average time between the onset of Alzheimer's disease and death is _____ years.

15. Genetic factors have been shown to play a role in dementia: **true   false**

16. Alzheimer's disease has been linked to what birth defect? _____.

17. Alzheimer's disease may involve dysfunction of the _____ system.

18. There is a controversial link between Alzheimer's disease and levels of what metal in the water system? _____

19. While there do not appear to be differences between men and women with regard to the overall prevalence of dementia, men appear to be at high risk for the _____ type and women are at higher risk for developing the _____ type.

20. The _____ test is used to assess planning problems and apraxia and is used to screen for dementia.

21. Patients with dementia benefit from _____ environments.

22. Patients with dementia who remain active have less _____.

23. Dementia with Lewy bodies show fluctuations in cognitive performance:
    true   false

24. Prevalence rates for dementia may be **lower** or **higher** in developing (as compared to developed) countries.

25. Elderly people who have been knocked unconscious as adults have a **higher** or **lower** risk of developing Alzheimer's disease.

Multiple Choice Questions

The following multiple choice questions will test your comprehension of the material presented in the chapter. Answers are listed at the end of the chapter.

1) All of the following are goals in designing an environment conducive to demented patients EXCEPT:

   a. keep the patients relatively inactive in order to prevent them from hurting themselves
   b. facilitate the patients knowledge of the environment through labeled rooms, hallways, etc.
   c. keep the environment negotiable (i.e., keep areas that a person will use often visible from their room if they cannot be remembered)
   d. stay abreast of safety and health issues

2) The _____ is probably the best known neuropsychological assessment procedure that involves the examination of performance on psychological tests to indicate whether a person has a brain disorder.

   a. Halstead-Reitan
   b. Weschler
   c. Symptoms Checklist-90 (SCL-90)
   d. Minnesota Multiphasic Personality Inventory-2 (MMPI-2)

3) _____ is a type of motor dysfunction that involves jerky, semi-purposeful movements of the person's face and limbs

   a. Anoxia   c. Chorea
   b. Myotonia   d. Lipofuscin

4) Which of the following appears to be the most common type of dementia?

   a. Pick's disease   c. Alzheimer's disease
   b. Huntington's disease   d. vascular dementia

5) All of the following are typical symptoms of Parkinson's disease EXCEPT:

   a. tremors   c. gradual dementia
   b. postural abnormalities   d. reduction in voluntary movements

6) A _____ deals primarily with diseases of the brain and the nervous system.

    a. neurologist
    b. psychiatrist
    c. psychologist
    d. cardiologist

7) Which of the following diagnoses depends on the presence of a positive family history for the disorder?

    a. Parkinson's disease
    b. Alzheimer's disease
    c. Pick's disease
    d. Huntington's disease

8) According to Baltes, _____ is to fluid intelligence as _____ is to crystallized intelligence.

    a. wisdom; knowledge
    b. knowledge; wisdom
    c. cognitive mechanics; cognitive pragmatics
    d. cognitive pragmatics; cognitive mechanics

9) The DSM-IV-TR currently classifies dementia and related clinical phenomena as:

    a. organic mental disorders
    b. biological mental disorders
    c. psychological disorders with organic aetiology
    d. cognitive disorders

10) Betty's physician handed her a hairbrush and said "Show me what you do with this object." She took the brush and brushed her hair with it, but was unable to name the object. She is most likely suffering from which of the following?

    a. agnosia
    b. aphasia
    c. apraxia
    d. ataxia

11) Hallucinations and delusions are seen in about _____ of dementia cases.

    a. 10 percent
    b. 20 percent
    c. 30 percent
    d. 40 percent

12) The most effective form of treatment for improving cognitive functioning in dementia of the Alzheimer's type is:

    a. cognitive therapy
    b. cognitive-behavioural therapy
    c. rational-emotive therapy (RET)
    d. no form of treatment is presently capable of improving cognitive functioning in dementia of the Alzheimer's type

13) One theory regarding Korsakoff's syndrome suggests that lack of _____ leads to atrophy of the medial thalamus.

a. zinc

b. vitamin C

c. vitamin B1 (thiamin)

d. potassium

14) Which of the following is a confusional state that develops over a short period of time and is often associated with agitation and hyperactivity?

a. delirium

b. amnesia

c. dementia

d. Alzheimer's disease

15) All of the following are frequently associated with dementia EXCEPT:

a. personality changes

b. emotional difficulties

c. high frequency of drug abuse

d. motivational problems

16) A definite diagnosis of Alzheimer's disease requires the observation of:

a. neurofibrillary tangles and senile plaques

b. degeneration of the substantia nigra

c. enlargement of the hypothalamus

d. all of the above

17) Dementia with Lewy bodies is NOT associated with:

a. hallucinations

b. variations in performance

c. a slow, gradual course

d. muscular rigidity

18) In order to qualify for a diagnosis of dementia, the person must exhibit memory impairment and which of the following?

a. aggressive behaviour

b. problems in abstract thinking

c. a previous episode of delirium

d. age of at least 65 years

19) All of the following are true of delirium EXCEPT:

a. it usually has a rapid onset

b. speech is typically confused

c. the person usually remains alert and responsive to the environment

d. it can be resolved

20) Parkinson's disease is primarily a disorder of the motor system that is caused by a loss of the neurotransmitter dopamine and a degeneration of this specific area of the brain stem:

a. substantia nigra

b. thalamus

c. fomix

d. superior colliculi

21) The incidence of dementia will be much greater in the near future because:

a. diagnostic criteria are more loosely defined
b. the average age of the population is increasing steadily
c. more people are being exposed to the environmental factors that have been shown to cause dementia
d. dementia is now striking people at a much earlier age

22) Which of the following can be distinguished from other types of dementia listed in the DSM-IV on the basis of speed of onset (i.e., cognitive impairment appears gradually, and the person's cognitive deterioration is progressive)?

a. vascular dementia
b. Huntington's disease
c. Alzheimer's disease
d. substance-induced persisting dementia

23) Which of the following is an example of a differentiated dementia?

a. Huntington's disease
b. Alzheimer's disease
c. vascular dementia
d. HIV disease

24) Some studies have confirmed an association between Alzheimer's disease and which of the following:

a. dependent personality disorder
b. vascular dementia
c. Korsakoff's syndrome
d. Down syndrome

25) _____ is a disorder that is frequently associated with dementia.

a. Bipolar disorder
b. Depression
c. Schizophrenia
d. Multiple personality disorder

26) Which of the following is/are treatment options for demented patients?

a. behavioural strategies
b. cognitive strategies
c. insight-oriented strategies
d. all of the above

27) All of the following are true of delirium EXCEPT:

a. it typically fluctuates throughout the day and is usually worse at night
b. the delirious person loses the ability to learn new information or becomes unable to recall previously learned information
c. the delirious person is likely to be disoriented with relation to time or place
d. the primary symptom is clouding of consciousness, which might also be described as a person's reduced awareness of his or her surroundings

Understanding Research — Fill in the Blank

Genetic Linkage Analysis: The text discusses this type of research in the Research Methods section. Finding the answers to these questions will help you get a good understanding of these issues.

1. Huntington's disease is considered an _____ because exactly _____ percent of an affected person's first-degree relatives will develop the disorder. Genetic linkage is shown between the gene causing the disorder and the locus for a _____ gene that is very close to it. Research was slow until the discovery of _____. What country did the family come from that had abnormally high levels of Huntington's disease and researchers studying them discovered a marker for the disease?

    _____

Brief Essay

As a final exercise, write out answers to the following brief essay questions. Then compare your answers with the material presented in the test.

    After you have answered these questions, review the "critical thinking" questions that are presented at the end of the text chapter. Answering these questions will help you integrate important issues and themes that have been featured throughout the chapter.

1. Briefly discuss how the behavioural effects of a stroke are different from those of dementia.

2. Discuss the environmental factors that have been shown to be possibly linked to some types of dementia. What do you see as being problematic with these findings? What must we be cautious of when interpreting this data?

3. Briefly discuss the similarities and differences between dementia and depression. Discuss a case where it might be difficult to distinguish them apart. How could this be done?

4. Briefly review the defining characteristics of delirium, Korsakoff's syndrome, Alzheimer's disease, and Huntington's disease.

Answer Key

Key Terms — Matching #1

1. a	7. n	13. c
2. i	8. f	14. k
3. o	9. e	15. q
4. l	10. j	16. h
5. p	11. m	17. g
6. b	12. d	

Key Terms — Matching #2

a. 5	d. 7	g. 15	j. 13	m. 16	p. 3
b. 14	e. 2	h. 10	k. 8	n. 11	q. 9
c. 4	f. 6	i. 17	l. 1	o. 12	

Review of Concepts

1. true
2. false
3. false
4. false
5. mechanics
6. true
7. 20 percent
8. vitamin
9. undifferentiated
10. death
11. a gene
12. unilateral
13. 8 percent
14. eight
15. true
16. Down Syndrome
17. immune
18. aluminum
19. vascular; Alzheimer's
20. The Clock Test
21. structured
22. depression
23. true
24. lower
25. higher

Multiple Choice

1. a	7. d	13. c	19. c	25. b
2. a	8. c	14. a	20. a	26. d
3. c	9. d	15. c	21. b	27. b
4. c	10. b	16. d	22. c	
5. c	11. b	17. c	23. a	
6. a	12. d	18. b	24. d	

Understanding Research

1. autosomal dominant trait; 50 percent; known; RFLPs; Venezuela

CHAPTER 15
MENTAL RETARDATION AND
PERVASIVE DEVELOPMENTAL DISORDERS

Chapter Outline

I.   Overview

II. Mental Retardation
    A. Typical Symptoms and Associated Features
       1. Significantly Subaverage IQ
         a. Measurement of Intelligence
         b. Controversies About Intelligence Tests
       2. Limitations in Adaptive Skills
       3. Onset Before Age 18 Years
    B. Classification
       1. Brief Historical Perspective
       2. Contemporary Classification
    C. Epidemiology
    D. Aetiological Considerations and Research
       1. Biological Factors
         a. Chromosomal Disorders
         b. Genetic Disorders
         c. Infectious Diseases
         d. Toxins
         e. Other Biological Abnormalities
         f. Normal Genetic Variation
       2. Psychological Factors
       3. Social Factors
    E. Treatment: Prevention and Normalisation
       1. Primary Prevention
       2. Secondary Prevention
       3. Tertiary Prevention
       4. Normalisation

III. Autistic Disorder and Pervasive Development Disorders
    A. Typical Symptoms and Associated Features
       1. Impaired Social Interaction
       2. Impaired Communication
       3. Stereotyped Behaviour, Interests, and Activities
       4. Apparent Sensory Deficits
       5. Self-injury
       6. Savant Performance

B. Classification
  1. Brief Historical Perspective
  2. Contemporary Classification
C. Epidemiology
D. Aetiological Considerations and Research
  1. Psychological and Social Factors
  2. Biological Factors
    a. Autism as a Consequence of Known Biological Disorders
    b. A Strongly Genetic Disorder?
    c. Integration: Multiple Pathways to a Brain Disorder
    d. Neurophysiology and Autism
    e. Neuroanatomy and Autism
    f. A Disorder of Brain Development
E. Treatment
  1. Course and Outcome
  2. Medication
  3. Facilitated Communication
  4. Psychotherapy: Intensive Behaviour Modification

Learning Objectives

After reviewing the material presented in this chapter, you should be able to:

1. Know the basic defining characteristics of mental retardation and autism.

2. Distinguish between practical intelligence and social intelligence.

3. Identify the four levels of mental retardation that DSM-IV delineates: mild, moderate, severe, and profound.

4. Appreciate that mental retardation can be caused by a variety of biological factors: chromosomal disorders, genetic disorders, infectious diseases, and environmental or chemical toxins.

5. Distinguish between primary, secondary, and tertiary prevention in treatment of mental retardation.

6. Describe the types of difficulties autistic children have with social interactions.

7. Define: dysprosody, echolalia, and pronoun rehearsal as they apply to impaired communication in autism.

8. Know the basic epidemiological statistics for autism.

9. Provide five reasons that we now believe autism is a biologically-based disorder.

10. Understand the advantages and disadvantages of intensive behaviour modification treatment for autism.

Key Terms — Matching #1

The following terms related to mental retardation and pervasive developmental disorders are important to know. To test your knowledge, match the following terms with their definitions. Answers are listed at the end of the chapter.

a. Mental retardation
b. Intelligence quotient (IQ)
c. Normal distribution
d. Standard deviation
e. Mild mental retardation
f. Moderate mental retardation
g. Severe mental retardation
h. Profound mental retardation
i. Down syndrome
j. Fragile-X syndrome
k. Klinefelter syndrome
l. XYY syndrome
m. Turner syndrome

n. Phenylketonuria (PKU)
o. Tuberous sclerosis
p. Tay-Sachs disease
q. Hurler syndrome
r. Lesch-Nyhan syndrome
s. Cytomegalovirus
t. Toxoplasmosis
u. Rubella
v. Syphillis
w. Genital herpes
x. Encephalitis
y. Meningitis
z. Foetal alcohol syndrome

1. ____ an infection of the membranes that line the brain which can lead to inflammation that can damage the brain
2. ____ a relatively common and usually harmless infection that can be passed to the foetus that can cause mental retardation
3. ____ a chromosomal abnormality transmitted genetically which sometimes leads to mental retardation or learning disabilities
4. ____ characterised by mental retardation and self-mutilation
5. ____ substantial limitations in present functioning characterised by significantly subaverage intellectual functioning, concurrent limitations in adaptive skills, and an onset before age 18
6. ____ motor skills, communication, and self-care are severely limited; constant supervision required
7. ____ a bacterial sexually transmitted disease which, if untreated, can be passed to the foetus and can result in physical and sensory handicaps in the foetus, including mental retardation
8. ____ a protozoan infection caused by ingestion of infected raw meats or from contact with infected cat feces which can cause brain damage to a foetus
9. ____ an intelligence test's rating of an individual's intellectual ability
10. ____ can generally function at the second grade level academically, require close training and supervision in work activities, and need family or group home supervision

11. ____ a very rare dominant-gene disorder characterised by white growths in the ventricles of the brain
12. ____ also called German measles, a viral infection that can cause severe mental retardation or death in a foetus
13. ____ caused by a recessive gene, this disorder involves the absence of an enzyme that metabolizes phenylalanine, an amino acid in certain foods, which leads to brain damage that results in mental retardation
14. ____ once thought to increase criminality but now recognised to be linked with social deviance and a mean IQ 10 points lower than average
15. ____ a measure of dispersion of scores around the mean
16. ____ an extra X chromosome in males that leads to low normal to mildly mentally retarded intellectual functioning
17. ____ results in gross physical abnormalities, including dwarfism, humpback, bulging head, and clawlike hands
18. ____ a bell-shaped frequency distribution
19. ____ a rare recessive-gene disorder that eventually results in death during the infant or preschool years which is particularly common among Jews of Eastern European heritage
20. ____ can be transmitted to the baby at birth and cause mental retardation, blindness, or death
21. ____ a missing X chromosome in females that leads to failure to develop sexually and intelligence near or within the normal range
22. ____ a disorder characterised by retarded physical development, a small head, narrow eyes, cardiac defects, and cognitive impairment
23. ____ can generally function at the sixth grade level academically, acquire vocational skills, and live in the community without special supports
24. ____ typically have abnormal motor development, sharply limited communicative speech, and require close supervision for community living
25. ____ a brain infection that can cause permanent brain damage in about 20 percent of cases
26. ____ a chromosomal disorder characterised by a distinctively abnormal physical appearance and mental retardation typically in the moderate to severe range

Key Terms — Matching #2

The following terms related to mental retardation and pervasive developmental disorders are important to know. To test your knowledge, match the following terms with their definitions. Answers are listed at the end of the chapter.

1. Mercury poisoning
2. Lead poisoning
3. Rh incompatibility
4. Premature birth

5. Anoxia
6. Epilepsy
7. Cultural-familial retardation
8. Heritability ratios

9. Reaction range
10. Amniocentesis
11. Normalisation
12. Mainstreaming
13. Pervasive developmental disorders
14. Autism
15. Gaze aversion
16. Dysprosody
17. Echolalia
18. Pronoun reversal
19. Self-stimulation
20. Apparent sensory deficit
21. Self-injurious behaviour
22. Savant performance
23. Asperger's disorder
24. Childhood disintegrative disorder
25. Rett's disorder

a. ＿＿＿ a diagnostic procedure in which fluid is extracted from the amniotic sac that protects the foetus during pregnancy and genetic tests are run on the fluid to identify genetic abnormalities

b. ＿＿＿ proposes that heredity determines the upper and lower limits of IQ, and experience determines the extent to which people reach their genetic potential

c. ＿＿＿ a person's repetition of phrases that are spoken to them

d. ＿＿＿ oxygen deprivation that can lead to brain damage

e. ＿＿＿ can produce severe physical, emotional, and intellectual impairments

f. ＿＿＿ disturbance in rate, rhythm, and intonation of speech production

g. ＿＿＿ indices to measure the extent of genetic contribution to a characteristic

h. ＿＿＿ a disorder similar to autism but which does not involve language delay

i. ＿＿＿ at least five months of normal development followed by a deceleration in head growth, loss of purposeful hand movements, loss of social engagement, poor coordination, and language delay

j. ＿＿＿ profound problems in social interaction, communication, and stereotyped behaviour, interests, and activities

k. ＿＿＿ confusion of pronouns, such as between "you" and "I"

l. ＿＿＿ active avoidance of eye contact

m. ＿＿＿ an exceptional ability in a highly specialised area of functioning

n. ＿＿＿ cases of mental retardation with no known aetiology that run in families and is linked with poverty

o. ＿＿＿ seizure disorder that can result in mental retardation

p. ＿＿＿ at toxic levels can produce behavioural and cognitive impairments, including mental retardation

q. ＿＿＿ means that people with mental retardation are entitled to live as much as possible like other members of society

r. ＿＿＿ unresponsiveness to auditory, tactile, or visual sensations even though there is no impairment in the sensory organ

s. ＿＿＿ unusual psychological problems that begin early in life and involve severe impairments in a number of areas of functioning

t. ＿＿＿ keeping mentally retarded children in regular classrooms as much as possible

u. ＿＿＿ problems in social interaction and communication, as well as stereotyped behaviour, with an onset following at least two years of normal development

v. ＿＿＿ poses a risk for subsequent pregnancies because the mother's body produces antibodies which attack the developing foetus unless treated with an antibiotic

w. ____ ritual actions such as flapping a string or spinning a top that seem to serve no other purpose than to provide sensory feedback

x. ____ can result in sensory impairments, poor physical development, and mental retardation; worse outcomes are typically associated with lower birth weights

y. ____ often repeated head-banging or biting of fingers

Names You Should Know — Matching

The following people have played an important role in research and theory of mental retardation and pervasive developmental disorders. To test your knowledge, match the following names with the descriptions of their contributions to the study of abnormal psychology. Answers are listed at the end of the chapter.

a. Alfred Binet   c. Langdon Down   e. Hans Asperger
b. Jean Marc Itard   d. Leo Kanner   f. O. Ivar Lovaas

1. ____ first described autism
2. ____ first described a subgroup of children with a chromosomal disorder later named after him
3. ____ described a subgroup of people with a disorder similar to autism but not involving mental retardation
4. ____ worked extensively with a feral child found living in the woods
5. ____ developed the first successful IQ test
6. ____ applied behavioural techniques to the management of people with autism

Review of Concepts — Fill in the Blank and True/False

This section will help focus your studying by testing whether you understand the concepts presented in the text. After you have read and reviewed the material, test your comprehension and memory by filling in the following blanks or circling the right answer. Answers are listed at the end of the chapter.

1. Which type of disorder is more common: **mental retardation   pervasive developmental disorders**

2. Intelligence is _____ distributed in the general population.

3. Intelligence tests have a mean of _____ and a standard deviation of_____.

4. The IQ of a particular person changes a lot over time: **true   false**

5. IQ tests measure potential for _____.

6. Adaptive skills include both _____ and _____ intelligence.

7. The physician who worked with Victor, the feral child of Aveyron, France, had great success in educating and socialising him: **true   false**

8. More people fall into the   **lower**   or   **upper**   range of the curve of IQs than would be predicted by a normal distribution.

9. What are the two categories of aetiology of mental retardation? _____ and _____

10. The incidence of Down syndrome is related to maternal and paternal _____.

11. Intensive intervention with people with Down syndrome has been shown to be beneficial to their achievement: **true   false**

12. People with Down syndrome typically die in their forties: **true   false**

13. Fragile-X syndrome is more likely to lead to mental retardation in boys than in girls: **true   false**

14. There is no known treatment for phenylketonuria: **true   false**

15. Pregnant women who drink one ounce of alcohol per day or less are not putting their foetus at risk for foetal alcohol syndrome: **true   false**

16. Crack babies are more likely to be born _____.

17. Children living in dilapidated housing are at increased risk for ingesting paint chips containing _____.

18. Rh incompatibility is only a potential danger to children of mothers who are Rh   **negative**   or   **positive**

19. The IQs of adopted children are more highly correlated to the IQs of their   **adoptive**   or   **biological**   parents.

20. What percentage of Canadian children under the age of 14 live in poverty? _____.

21. Environment has been shown to have little effect on IQ: **true   false**

22. Children who participate in Head Start are less likely to _____.

23. The use of neuroleptics to manage aggression and uncontrolled behaviour among mentally retarded patients in institutions is recommended: **true**   **false**

24. People with autism have unusual physical appearances: **true**   **false**

25. Autism is not usually identified until the child reaches kindergarten: **true**   **false**

26. Children with autism tend to be very affectionate: **true**   **false**

27. Many children with autism remain mute: **true**   **false**

28. People with autism have problems in their capacity for social _____.

29. People with autism   **resist**   or   **require**   routine.

30. People with autism have superior intelligence: **true**   **false**

31. Some brain injured patients demonstrate savant abilities: **true**   **false**

32. Autism is more common among the upper social classes: **true**   **false**

33. Autism is more common among   **boys**   or   **girls**

34. Siblings of people with autism are likely to have autism: **true**   **false**

35. Autism is likely caused by some combination of poor parenting and biological factors:
    true   **false**

36. MZ twins show higher concordance for autism than DZ twins: **true**   **false**

37. Most people grow out of autism: **true**   **false**

38. A number of teens with autism develop _____ disorders.

39. A number of medications show promise in improving functioning of autistic patients: **true**   **false**

40. Behavioural treatments to reduce self-injurious behaviour in autistic patients are controversial because they involve _____.

41. The only form of treatment found to be effective in increasing the functioning of autistic patients is _____ operant behaviour therapy.

42. Facilitated Communication has been shown to be an effective treatment for autism:
    true   **false**

Multiple Choice Questions

The following multiple choice questions will test your comprehension of the material presented in the chapter. Answers are listed at the end of the chapter.

1) Which of the following toxins presents the greatest threat to a foetus?

   a. cigarettes
   b. alcohol

   c. lead
   d. mercury

2) All of the following are central symptoms of autism EXCEPT:

   a. impaired communication abilities
   b. impairments in social interaction
   c. abnormalities of the eyes, nose, and ears
   d. stereotyped patterns of behaviour, interests, and activities

3) Mild mental retardation is designated for individual with IQ scores between which of the following?

   a. 20–25 and 40
   b. 35–40 and 50

   c. 50-55 and 70
   d. 65-70 and 90

4) As outlined in your text, which of the following has been suggested as an interpretation for pronoun reversal as documented in some cases of autism?

   a. pronoun reversal demonstrates a lack of understanding of speech
   b. pronoun reversal is a result of faulty neurotransmitters
   c. pronoun reversal results from damage to specific areas in the frontal lobe
   d. pronoun reversal is due to the autistic child's disinterest in other people

5) Autism is considered to be a _____ disorder, with approximately _____ out of every 10,000 children qualifying for the diagnosis.

   a. rare; 4–5
   b. rare; 20–25

   c. common; 1,000-1,500
   d. common; 3,000-3,500

6) Which of the following is one of the most important current secondary prevention efforts in preventing cultural-familial retardation?

   a. amniocentesis
   b. prenatal care

   c. Head Start
   d. rare; 20-25

7) Treatment for self-injurious behaviour that is sometimes seen in autistic children is controversial because:

a. there is no empirical support to back up the treatment
b. the treatment typically involves punishment (e.g., slap or mild electric shock)
c. the treatment has been relatively ineffective
d. the treatment has been used without guardian consent

8) The reaction range concept of IQ proposed that (the) _____ determines the upper and lower limits of IQ, and (the) _____ determines the extent to which people fulfill their genetic potential.

a. heredity; experience
b. experience; heredity
c. parents' IQ; age
d. age; parents' IQ

9) Mental retardation with a specific, known organic cause:

a. is typically more common among families living in poverty
b. generally is more common among Hispanics and African-Americans
c. is most prevalent among the upper class
d. generally has an equal prevalence among all social classes

10) Which of the following was the original developer of IQ tests?

a. Douglas Biklin
b. Alfred Binet
c. Leo Kanner
d. O. Ivan Lovaas

11) All of the following are true of autistic children EXCEPT:

a. most are normal in physical appearance
b. physical growth and development is generally normal
c. their body movements are typically grossly uncoordinated
d. they sometimes have unusual actions and postures

12) Premature birth is defined either as a birth weight of less than 2.5 kg or as birth before _____weeks of gestation.

a. 35
b. 36
c. 37
d. 38

13) The most common form of self-injury that can accompany autism and other pervasive developmental disorders is:

a. head-banging
b. repetitive hitting of objects with one's fists
c. dare-devil behaviours (i.e., skydiving, bungee jumping, etc.)
d. cutting of oneself with sharp objects

14) All of the following are diagnostic criteria for autism EXCEPT:

    a. lack of social or emotional reciprocity
    b. a prior diagnosis of Rett's disorder
    c. apparently compulsive adherence to specific, nonfunctional routines or rituals
    d. lack of varied spontaneous make-believe play or social imitative play appropriate to developmental level

15) Autism is believed to be caused by:

    a. poor parenting
    b. an abusive environment
    c. neurological abnormalities
    d. there is no known etiology for autism

16) Approximately _____ of children in Canada are born to adolescent mothers.

    a. 8 percent   c. 11–17 percent
    b. 2–5 percent   d. 20 percent

17) Savant performance is NOT typical in which of the following areas:

    a. artistic   c. musical
    b. mathematical   d. athletic

18) Which of the following interpretations of self-stimulation is most plausible according to your text?

    a. it is a way for the autistic child to feel like he or she is similar to others
    b. it serves the purpose of increasing stimulation to the autistic child who receives too little sensory input
    c. it serves the function of making a terrifying world more constant and predictable and therefore less frightening
    d. it is merely a repetitive behaviour that serves no function

19) According to the American Association of Mental Retardation's (AAMR) definition, mental retardation manifests before age:

    a. 5   c. 13
    b. 8   d. 18

20) Which of the following is an infectious disease that is the result of infection of the brain and produces inflammation and permanent damage in approximately 20 percent of all cases?

    a. meningitis   c. encephalitis
    b. rubella   d. cytomegalovirus

21) Which of the following is caused by the presence of an extra chromosome and is characterised by a distinctively abnormal physical appearance, which includes slanting eyes, small head and stature, protruding tongue, and a variety of organ, muscle, and skeletal abnormalities?

a. Down syndrome
b. Foetal Alcohol syndrome
c. Phenylketonuria (PKU)
d. Tuberous sclerosis

22) Severe mental retardation accounts for approximately _____ of the mentally retarded.

a. 1–2 percent
b. 3–4 percent
c. 8–10 percent
d. 12–15 percent

23) Which of the following is the most promising approach to treating autism?

a. intensive behaviour modification using operant conditioning techniques
b. antidepressant medication
c. psychodynamic therapy that focuses on providing a nurturing, supportive environment
d. none of the above have been effective in treating autism

24) Both mental retardation and pervasive developmental disorders include all of the following EXCEPT:

a. either are present at birth or begin early in life
b. serious disruptions in many areas of functioning, often including an inability to care for oneself independently
c. gross physical abnormalities
d. often, but not always, associated with a below-average IQ

25) Autism is usually first noticed:

a. early in life
b. during the teenage years
c. in adulthood
d. late in life

26) Which of the following terms was used for several years to classify autism together with other severe forms of childhood psychopathology?

a. childhood dissociation
b. disruptive childhood behaviours
c. psychopathology first evident in childhood
d. childhood schizophrenia

27) Which of the following developmental periods is particularly important to the course of autism?

a. birth to 6 months
b. 6-36 months

c. early school years
d. early adulthood

28) Allen is a six-year-old boy who has been diagnosed with autism. Frequently, when asked "would you like a drink," Allen will repeat the question over and over again. This is an example of:

a. pronoun reversal
b. dysprosody

c. echolalia
d. self-stimulation

Understanding Research — Fill in the Blank

Central Tendency, Variability, and Standard Scores: The text discusses these statistical issues in the Research Methods section. Finding the answers to these questions will help you get a good understanding of these issues.

1. A frequency distribution is _____
    _____. The
    mean is the _____ of a distribution of scores, a measure
    of central _____. The median is the _____
    of a frequency distribution. The mode is _____ _____ in
    a distribution.

2. The range is a simple measure of _____. Variability gives an indi-
    cation of how much the scores vary, or are dispersed around the mean. Why are
    the differences from the mean squared when calculating the variance?
    _____ Why is
    the standard deviation used more often than the variance?
    _____ Z-scores
    have a mean of _____ and a standard deviation of _____.

Brief Essay

As a final exercise, write out answers to the following brief essay questions. Then compare your answers with the material presented in the text.

After you have answered these questions, review the "critical thinking" questions that are presented at the end of the text chapter. Answering these questions will help you integrate important issues and themes that have been featured throughout the chapter.

1. Despite the value of IQ tests in predicting academic performance, one controversial question is whether intelligence tests are "culture fair." Briefly discuss your views on this topic, including material from your chapter to support your ideas.

2. Currently, mental retardation can be classified according to the American Association on Mental Retardation (AAMR) and by the DSM-IV. Briefly discuss the similarities and differences in classification according to these two approaches.

3. Briefly discuss the various aetiological considerations regarding autism. Which hypotheses seem most plausible to you and why? What research supports these hypotheses?

4. Briefly review the literature on facilitated communication as a treatment for autism.

5. Briefly discuss the ethical debate regarding behaviour modification treatments for decreasing potentially dangerous behaviours in autistic children. Do you believe these treatments to be unethical? If so, what do you believe are some viable options?

6. Briefly review the history of the sexual sterilisation and eugenics movement in Canada.

Answer Key

Key Terms — Matching #1

1. y	10. f	19. p
2. s	11. o	20. w
3. j	12. u	21. m
4. r	13. n	22. z
5. a	14. l	23. e
6. h	15. d	24. g
7. v	16. k	25. x
8. t	17. q	26. i
9. b	18. c	

Names You Should Know

1. d
2. c
3. e
4. b
5. a
6. f

Key Terms — Matching #2

a. 10	d. 5	g. 8	j. 14	m. 22
b. 9	e. 1	h. 23	k. 18	n. 7
C. 17	f. 16	i. 25	l. 15	o. 6

p. 2   r. 20   t. 12   v. 3   x. 4
q. 11   s. 13   u. 24   w. 19   y. 21

Multiple Choice

1. b	7. b	13. a	19. d	25. a
2. c	8. a	14. b	20. c	26. d
3. c	9. d	15. c	21. a	27. c
4. a	10. b	16. a	22. b	28. c
5. a	11. c	17. d	23. a	
6. c	12. d	18. c	24. c	

Review of Concepts

1. mental retardation
2. normally
3. 100; 15
4. false
5. school achievement
6. practical; social
7. false
8. lower
9. organic; familial
10. age
11. true
12. true
13. true
14. false
15. false
16. premature
17. lead
18. negative
19. biological
20. 30%
21. false

22. repeat a grade
23. false
24. false
25. false
26. false
27. true
28. imitation
29. require
30. false
31. true
32. false
33. boys
34. true
35. false
36. true
37. false
38. seizure
39. false
40. punishment
41. intensive
42. false

Understanding Research

1. a way of arranging data according to the frequencies of different possible scores; arithmetic average; tendency; midpoint; the most frequent score

2. variability; to keep them from summing to zero; because it is in the original units of measurement; zero; one

CHAPTER 16
PSYCHOLOGICAL DISORDERS OF CHILDHOOD

Chapter Outline

I. Overview

II. Externalising Disorders
    A. Typical Symptoms of Externalising Disorders
        1. Rule Violations
            a. Serious Rule Violations
            b. Children's Age and Rule Violations
        2. Negativity, Anger, and Aggression
        3. Impulsivity
        4. Hyperactivity
        5. Attention deficits
    B. Classification of Externalising Disorders
        1. Brief Historical Perspective
            a. Attention-Deficit Hyperactivity Disorder
            b. Oppositional Defiant Disorder
            c. ADHD versus ODD
            d. Subtypes of ADHD
            e. Conduct Disorder
    C. Epidemiology of Externalising Disorders
        1. Family Risk Factors
    D. Aetiology of Externalising Disorders
        1. Biological Factors
            a. Temperament
            b. Genetics
            c. Neuropsychological Abnormalities
            d. Food Additives and Sugar
        2. Social Factors
            a. Parenting Styles
            b. Coercion
            c. Love and Discipline
            d. Conflict and Inconsistent Discipline
            e. Broader Social Influences: Peers, Neighbourhoods, Television and Society
            f. Social Factors in Attention-Deficit Hyperactivity Disorder
        3. Psychological Factors
        4. Integration and Alternative Pathways
    E. Treatment of Externalising Disorders
        1. Psychostimulants and ADHD
            a. The "Paradoxical Effect" Paradox
            b. Usage and Effects

c. Side Effects
d. Antidepressant Medication for ADHD
2. Behavioural Family Therapy
3. Treatment of Conduct Disorders and Juvenile Delinquency
a. Residential Programs and Juvenile Courts

III. Internalising and Other Disorders
A. Typical Symptoms of Internalising and Other Disorders
1. Depressive Symptoms
2. Children's Fears and Anxiety
3. Separation Anxiety Disorder and School Refusal
4. Troubled Peer Relationships
5. Specific Developmental Deviations
B. Classification of Internalising and Other Disorders
1. Brief Historical Perspective
2. DSM-IV and DSM-IV-TR: Strengths and Weaknesses
a. Overinclusive Listing of Disorders
b. Contextual Classifications?
C. Epidemiology of Internalising and Other Disorders
1. Suicide
D. Aetiology of Internalising and Other Disorders
1. Biological Factors
2. Social Factors: A Focus on Attachments
a. Reactive Attachment Disorder
b. Insecure Attachments
c. Separation and Loss
3. Psychological Factors
E. Treatment of Internalising Disorders
1. Course and Outcome

Learning Objectives

After reviewing the material presented in this chapter, you should be able to:

1. Distinguish between externalisin and internalising disorders of childhood.

2. State some of the primary factors considered in the evaluation of externalising symptoms.

3. Compare separation anxiety with separation anxiety disorder.

4. Understand that children's psychological problems are not simply miniature versions of adult disorders.

5. Describe some of the rare childhood disorders: pica, rumination disorder, Tourette's disorder, selective autism, reactive attachment disorder, Stereotypic movement disorder, encopresis, and enuresis.

6. Give the defining characteristics of conduct disorder, oppositional defiant disorder, and attention-deficit/hyperactivity disorder.

7. Understand how attachment theory attempts to explain disorders of childhood.

8. State and describe the four parenting styles and explain how inconsistent parenting leads to externalising symptoms in children.

9. List and describe some of the genetic and biological evidence, both positive and negative, concerning the aetiology of childhood disorders.

10. Describe the ways in which behavioural family therapy is utilised in the treatment of externalising disorders.

11. Identify the common course and outcome of the primary childhood disorders.

Key Terms — Matching #1

The following terms related to psychological disorders of childhood are important to know. To test your knowledge, match the following terms with their definitions. Answers are listed at the end of the chapter.

a. Externalising disorders
b. Attention deficit-hyperactivity disorder
c. Oppositional-defiant disorder
d. Conduct disorder
e. Internalising disorders
f. Learning disorders
g. Continuous performance test
h. Separation anxiety
i. Separation anxiety disorder
j. School refusal
k. Peer sociometrics
l. Pica
m. Rumination disorder

n. Tourette's disorder
o. Stereotypic movement disorder
p. Selective autism
q. Reactive attachment disorder
r. Encopresis
s. Enuresis
t. Hyperkinesis
u. sustained attention
v. Juvenile delinquency
w. "Paradoxical effects" of drugs
x. Representative sample
y. Attachment theory
z. Anaclitic depression

1. _____ a particular attentional problem involving difficulty staying on task
2. _____ consistent failure to speak in certain social situations, while speech is unrestricted in other situations
3. _____ a set of proposals about the normal development of attachments and the adverse consequences of troubled attachment relationships
4. _____ a legal classification determined by a judge
5. _____ a disorder of childhood characterised by persistent and excessive worry for the safety of an attachment figure, fears of separation, nightmares with separation themes, and refusal to be alone

6. ____ an outdated term for hyperactivity
7. ____ the lack of social responsiveness found among infants who do not have a consistent attachment figure
8. ____ normal distress following separation from an attachment figure which peaks at about 15 months of age
9. ____ repeated motor and verbal tics
10. ____ when the effects of a drug on a target population are opposite to the effects of that same drug on a normal population
11. ____ an empirically derived category of disruptive child behaviour problems that create problems for the external world
12. ____ the repeated regurgitation and rechewing of food
13. ____ a disorder defined primarily by behaviour that is illegal as well as antisocial
14. ____ characterised by severely disturbed and developmentally inappropriate social relationships
15. ____ a sample that accurately represents some larger group of people
16. ____ an extreme reluctance to go to school, accompanied by symptoms of anxiety
17. ____ a laboratory task that requires the subject to monitor and respond to numbers or letters presented on a computer screen
18. ____ a group of educational problems characterised by academic performance that is notably below academic aptitude
19. ____ a method of assessing children's social relationships and categorising children's social standing by obtaining information on who is "liked most" and who is "liked least" from a group of children who know each other
20. ____ self-stimulation or self-injurious behaviour that is serious enough to require treatment
21. ____ inappropriately controlled defecation
22. ____ a disorder characterised by hyperactivity, inattention, and impulsivity
23. ____ the persistent eating of nonnutritive substances
24. ____ inappropriately controlled urination
25. _____ a disorder characterised by negative, hostile, and defiant behaviour
26. ____ an empirically derived category of psychological problems of childhood that affect the child more than the external world

Key Terms — Matching #2

The following terms related to psychological disorders of childhood are important to know. To test your knowledge, match the following terms with their definitions. Answers are listed at the end of the chapter.

1. Secure attachments
2. Anxious attachments
3. Anxious avoidant attachments
4. Anxious resistant attachments
5. Disorganized attachments

6. Resilience
7. Authoritative parenting
8. Authoritarian parenting
9. Indulgent parenting
10. Neglectful parenting

11. Coercion
12. Time-out
13. Temperament
14. Salicylates
15. Delay of gratification
16. Emotion regulation
17. Psychostimulants
18. Dose-response effects
19. Behavioural family therapy

20. Parent training
21. Negotiation
22. Multisystemic therapy
23. Recidivism
24. Rehabilitation
25. Parens patrial
26. Diversion
27. Problem-solving skills training

a. ____ an anxious attachment where the infant is wary of exploration, not easily soothed by the attachment figure, and angry or ambivalent about contact

b. ____ an anxious attachment where the infant responds inconsistently because of conflicting feelings toward an inconsistent caregiver who is the potential source of either reassurance or fear

c. ____ a food additive that was thought to be related to ADHD but which controlled research has found to be unrelated

d. ____ the response to different dosages of medications

e. ____ parenting that is unconcerned with both the child's emotional needs and needs for discipline

f. ____ repeat offending

g. ____ learning to identify, evaluate, and control one's feelings based on the reactions, attitudes, and advice of others in the social world

h. ____ combines family treatment with coordinated interventions in other important contexts of the troubled child's life

i. ____ teaching parents discipline strategies

j. ____ parenting that is affectionate but lax in discipline

k. ____ parenting that is strict, often harsh and undemocratic, as well as lacking in warmth

l. ____ keeping problem youths out of the juvenile justice system

m. ____ a technique of briefly isolating a child following misbehaviour

n. ____ infants with these attachments are fearful about exploration and are not easily comforted by their attachment figures, who respond inadequately or inconsistently to the child's needs

o. ____ infants with these attachments separate easily and explore away from their attachment figure but seek comfort when threatened

p. ____ a child's inborn behavioural characteristics, such as activity level, emotionality, and sociability

q. ____ a form of family treatment which trains parents to use the principles of operant conditioning to improve child discipline

r. ____ a system of interaction in which parents and children reciprocally reinforce child misbehaviour and parent capitulation

s. ____ an anxious attachment where the infant is generally unwary of strange situations and shows little preference for the attachment figure over others

t. ____ the adaptive ability to defer smaller but immediate rewards for larger long-term benefits
u. ____ the goal of treatment for delinquent youths
v. ____ a process in which young people are actively involved in defining rules
w. ____ the ability to bounce back from adversity
x. ____ the state as parent
y. ____ medications used to treat children with ADHD
z. ____ parenting that is both loving and firm
aa. ____ a technique where children are taught to evaluate a problem and consider alternatives before acting

Names You Should Know — Matching

The following people have played an important role in research and theory of psychological disorders of childhood. To test your knowledge, match the following names with the descriptions of their contributions to the study of abnormal psychology. Answers are listed at the end of the chapter.

a. Mary Ainsworth   c. John Bowlby   e. Virginia Douglas
b. Michael Rutter   d. Lawrence Kohlberg   f. Benjamin Feingold

1. ____ developed the family adversity index
2. ____ conducted many empirical studies on attachment theory
3. ____ the first to recognise the importance of attentional problems in ADHD children
4. ____ proposed that food additives caused hyperactivity
5. ____ studied moral development in children
6. ____ developed attachment theory

Review of Concepts — Fill in the Blank and True/False

This section will help focus your studying by testing whether you understand the concepts presented in the text. After you have read and reviewed the material, test your comprehension and memory by filling in the following blanks or circling the right answer. Answers are listed at the end of the chapter.

1. Which of the following disorders involves violations of laws?

   oppositional defiant disorder   conduct disorder

2. It has been estimated that only 5 percent of juvenile offenders account for _____ percent of juvenile offenses.

   About 10 percent   about 30 percent   about 50 percent

3. Adult antisocial behaviour is better predicted by information about the person during **childhood** or **adolescence**.

4. In adolescence, violation of rules is _____.

5. Impulsivity is acting before _____.

6. Where is hyperactivity often first noticed? _____

7. The behavioural problems that characterise ADHD are largely **intentional** or **unintentional**.

8. Assessment of children's feelings is **straightforward** or **difficult**.

9. Parents are very good at detecting their children's depression: **true**   **false**

10. If in error, parents are likely to **overestimate** or **underestimate** their children's depression.

11. Fears in children are a symptom of some emotional disorder: **true**   **false**

12. School refusal often indicates a child's fear of _____.

13. Which category of peer ratings is the most correlated with psychological disorders?

_____

14. What type of norms are essential in assessing abnormal behaviour in children?

_____norms

15. A learning disorder is defined as one or two standard deviations between

_____ and _____.

16. There is a high degree of comorbidity between learning disorders and which two psychological disorders? _____ and _____

17. Learning disorders are easily treated: **true**   **false**

18. Encopresis and enuresis are usually **causes of** or **reactions to** psychological distress.

19. The bell and pad is a device that is effective in treating _____.

20. The current DSM-IV is probably **overinclusive** or **underinclusive** in its listing of childhood psychological disorders.

21. Hyperactivity is the result of inattention: **true** **false**

22. ADHD and oppositional defiant disorder are separate but _____ disorders.

23. More **boys** or **girls** are treated for psychological disorders; more **men** or **women** enter into therapy.

24. Girls are more likely to have _____ problems, and boys are more likely to have _____ problems.

25. Risk for _____ problems increase substantially when more than one family adversity risk factor is present.

26. What is the third leading cause of death among teenagers? _____

27. Picking up a crying infant makes it **easier** or **more difficult** to manage.

28. Children with serious conduct problems often have parents who use what type of parenting? _____

29. Negative attention is sometimes _____ to children.

30. Crime rates are about the same in the United States and in Europe: **true** **false**

31. Research has shown that critical and demanding parenting is the **cause** or **result** of hyperactive child behaviour.

32. A certain temperamental style has been linked to _____ disorders in adulthood.

33. Genetic factors appear to be strongly linked to ADHD: **true** **false**

34. Children with externalising disorders may be less_____reactive than other children.

35. Research has shown that sugar increases hyperactive behaviour: **true** **false**

36. Children with externalising disorder have problems with _____ control.

37. Aggressive children demonstrate immaturity in moral development: **true** **false**

38. Children with mothers who are depressed are more likely to develop _____.

39. Children usually grow out of internalising disorders: **true** **false**

40. Antidepressants are effective in treating children with depression: **true**   **false**

41. Psychostimulants are effective in treating children with ADHD: **true**   **false**

42. Psychostimulants have a paradoxical effect on children with ADHD, which demonstrates the biological underpinnings of the disorder: **true**   **false**

43. Psychostimulants are taken for a couple of weeks and their effects last for several months at a time: **true**   **false**

44. Psychostimulants given at high doses provide maximum _____ _____ but interfere with _____

45. Medication is more helpful in the treatment of ADHD than behavioural family therapy:
     true   **false**

46. When juveniles are diverted from the juvenile justice system, they show higher rates of recidivism: **true**   **falsee**

47. Psychostimulant use among preschoolers has significantly increased:
     true   **false**

Multiple Choice Questions
The following multiple choice questions will test your comprehension of the material presented in the chapter. Answers are listed at the end of the chapter.

1)   In his study on family adversity, Michael Rutter found that all of the following were predictors of behaviour problems among children EXCEPT:

   a. low income
   b. overcrowding in the home
   c. conflict between parents
   d. paternal depression

2)   All of the following are major problems in evaluating children's internalising symptoms EXCEPT:

   a. there are insufficient self-report measures to assess internalising symptoms in children
   b. it is much more difficult for adults to assess children's inner experiences than it is to observe children's behaviour
   c. children often are not reliable or valid informants about their internal life
   d. children's capacity to recognize emotions in themselves emerges slowly over the course of development and therefore they may not be aware of their own emotional turmoil

3) Reactive attachment disorder is most likely caused by which of the following?

    a. it appears to have genetic origins
    b. an unstable home environment in which caregivers are frequently changing
    c. extremely neglectful parenting
    d. its aetiology is unknown

4) All of the following are major subtypes of externalising disorders EXCEPT:

    a. attention-deficit/hyperactivity disorder
    b. conduct disorder
    c. depression
    d. oppositional defiant disorder

5) Which of the following is the most helpful information for scientists to have for predicting adult antisocial behaviour?

    a. information obtained during birth and infancy
    b. information obtained during childhood
    c. information obtained during adolescence
    d. information obtained during adulthood

6) According to a panel of experts assembled by the National Academy of Sciences, at least _____ percent of the 63 million children living in the United States suffer from a mental disorder:

    a. 5   c. 17
    b. 12   d. 23

7) Which of the following is a sample that accurately depicts a larger group of people?

    a. representative sample   c. convenience sample
    b. random sample   d. heterogeneous sample

8) _____ appears to have environmental origins, while _____ appears to have some sort of biological cause.

    a. Attention-deficit/hyperactivity disorder; oppositional defiant disorder
    b. Oppositional defiant disorder; attention-deficit/hyperactivity disorder
    c. Conduct disorder; oppositional defiant disorder
    d. Oppositional defiant disorder; conduct disorder

9) Separation anxiety disorder is typically associated with all of the following EXCEPT:

    a. fears of getting lost or being kidnapped
    b. refusal to be alone
    c. persistent and excessive worry for the safety of an attachment figure
    d. refusal to interact with others when the attachment figure is not present

10) Typically, the attachment figure for an infant with an anxious attachment responds to the infant in which of the following ways?

   a. appropriately attends to the infant's needs
   b. inadequately or inconsistently attends to the infant's needs
   c. immediately attends to the infant's needs
   d. is completely unresponsive to the infant's needs

11) Suicide is the second leading cause of death amongst Canadian Teenagers. Which group has shown the largest upward trend in suicide rates over the past decade?

   15 -19 year olds   c. 13 -15 year olds
   10 -12 year olds   d. 20 - 23 year olds

12) Which of the following is a well-known treatment device that awakens children with enuresis by setting off an alarm as they begin to wet the bed?

   a. bell and pad   c. sensitive signal seat
   b. light and alarm   d. responsive wetting device

13) Which of the following is characterised by self-stimulation or self-injurious behaviour?

   a. conduct disorder
   b. developmental coordination disorder
   c. Tourette's disorder
   d. stereotypic movement disorder

14) ADHD is characterised by all of the following symptoms EXCEPT:

   a. impulsivity   c. aggression
   b. hyperactivity   d. inattention

15) Treatment with children often begins with which of the following?

   a. an attempt to get the adults (i.e., parents, teachers) to agree as to what the problem really is
   b. identifying a disorder and then building hypotheses to either prove or disprove it
   c. helping the child to identify his or her problems
   d. an attempt to treat the family, independent of the child, in order to facilitate change in the child's environment

16) Which of the following gender differences is NOT TRUE with respect to internalising and externalising problems?

   a. more adult men enter into therapy than do adult women
   b. boys are treated more for psychological problems than are girls
   c. by early adult life, more females report psychological problems than males
   d. boys have far more externalising disorders than girls

17) According to the "peer sociometric method" of assessing children's relationships, which of the following groups is characterised by a high frequency of "liked least" ratings and a low frequency of "liked most" ratings?

    a. average
    b. neglected
    c. rejected
    d. controversial

18) All of the following are internalising symptoms EXCEPT:

    a. somatic complaints
    b. fears
    c. aggressive behaviour
    d. sadness

19) All of the following factors influence how adults evaluate children's rule violations EXCEPT:

    a. frequency of the child's behaviour
    b. duration of the child's behaviour
    c. intensity of the child's behaviour
    d. all of the above

20) Brandon is a three-year-old who frequently throws a tantrum when in the grocery store if he does not get what he wants. Because this is such an embarrassing situation for his mother, she will give Brandon whatever he desires in order to get his cooperation. In this case, Brandon is being _____ while his mother is being _____.

    a. positively reinforced; negatively reinforced
    b. negatively reinforced; positively reinforced
    c. classically conditioned; punished
    d. positively reinforced; punished

21) Infants typically develop a fear of _____ around the age of seven to eight months.

    a. strangers
    b. the dark
    c. monsters
    d. unfamiliar environments

22) Which of the following is the process of shaping children's behaviour and attitudes to conform to the expectations of parents, teachers, and society as a whole?

    a. modeling
    b. socialization
    c. conditioning
    d. vicarious learning

Understanding Research — Fill in the Blank

The Ontario Child Health Study: The text presents a detailed description of a study by David R. Offord and Michael H. Boyle. The OCHS is the largest epidemiological study of children in Canada, and one of the largest, most detailed studies of its kind in the world. The OCHS has provided valuable information about the prevalence, co-occurrence, risk factors, and long-term outcome of mental disorders. Finding the answers to these questions will help you get a good understanding of this study and why it is important. It is not necessary to memorize the answers; the process of finding them in the textbook will help you learn the material you need to know.

1. In this study, children between the ages of _____ were assessed on four dimensions of childhood problems that were previous identified as being common and causing considerable suffering to children and their families. The four childhood disorders were: _____, _____, _____, and

    _____.

2. Information about children was collected from a number of different sources, including: the _____ head of the house, _____ and youths between 12 and 16 years of age. Information about the child's use of health services and use of illicit substances was also collected.

3. Results revealed a high prevalence of disorders in children. _____ percent of children showed one of the four disorders in the past 6 months. Although the criteria for diagnosing a behavioural problem in a child were _____ stringent than those specified by the DSM-IV, the results of this study suggest that behavioural problems are very common in children.

4. Conduct disorder was more prevalent amongst _____, particularly the _____ ones; hyperactivity was more prevalent amongst _____, regardless of age. _____ was more common in older girls than older boys.

5. The OCHS also found a very high rate, _____ percent, of an additional diagnosis amongst those demonstrating behavioural or emotional problems. More specifically, co-morbidity most often occurred _____ the two clusters of disorders. Presence of one or more diagnoses was associated with _____ school performance, substance use, and _____ amongst the youth. Despite the fact that having one or more of the four diagnoses was associated with _____ use of mental health services, very few specialised mental health services actually reached the affected children.

6. Four year follow-up of these children indicated that conduct disorder remains stable for _____ of children who were diagnosed with conduct disorder four years earlier and that more than half of the children who were diagnosed with conduct disorder at follow-up _____ four years earlier. Two diagnoses were associated with substance use at follow-up: _____ and _____.

Samples and Sampling: The text discusses this research issue in the Research Methods section. Finding the answers to these questions will help you get a good understanding of these issues.

7. Instead of representative samples, researchers often use _____ samples in their research. Representative samples are essential only when trying to determine questions such as whether single parenting causes _____. What type of sample can be used to generalize to a larger sample? _____ In one of the most famous examples of sampling errors, newspaper headlines stated that _____ beat _____ in the presidential elections.

8. In a survey of _____ children that constituted a _____ sample, _____ percent of children had a learning, behavioural, or developmental disorder. _____ percent had significant emotional or behavioural problems. More than _____percent had received treatment for psychological problems. These problems were associated, but only modestly, with family _____. Black and Latino parents reported _____ problems with white parents, but when _____ records were examined, they had more problems.

Brief Essay

As a final exercise, write out answers to the following brief essay questions. Then compare your answers with the material presented in the text.

   After you have answered these questions, review the "critical thinking" questions that are presented at the end of the text chapter. Answering these questions will help you integrate important issues and themes that have been featured throughout the chapter.

1. Discuss the challenges of identifying internalising problems in children. How do different sources of information vary on their estimation of internalising problems (e.g., children, parents, teachers, self-report inventories)? What is the best course of action for psychologists and researchers studying these problems?

2. Your text discusses classifying children's psychological problems in the context of key interpersonal relationships rather than using the current method of classification. Briefly discuss the strengths and weaknesses of each approach.

3. Compare and contrast the following disorders: attention-deficit/hyperactivity disorder, oppositional defiant disorder, and conduct disorder. Include a brief discussion on the overlap between these disorders.

ANSWER KEY

Key Terms — Matching #1

1. u	10. w	19. k
2. p	11. a	20. o
3. y	12. m	21. r
4. v	13. d	22. b
5. i	14. q	23. l
6. t	15. x	24. s
7. z	16. j	25. c
8. h	17. g	26. e
9. n	18. f	

Names You Should Know

1. b
2. a
3. e
4. f
5. d
6. c

Key Terms — Matching #2

a. 4	j. 9	s. 3
b. 5	k. 8	t. 15
c. 14	l. 6	u. 24
d. 18	m. 12	v. 21
e. 10	n. 2	w. 6
f. 21	o. 1	x. 25
g. 16	p. 13	y. 17
h. 22	q. 19	z. 7
i. 20	r. 11	aa. 27

Multiple Choice

1. d	6. b	11. a	16. a	21. a
2. a	7. a	12. a	17. c	22. b
3. c	8. b	13. d	18. c	
4. c	9. d	14. c	19. d	
5. b	10. b	15. a	20. a	

Review of Concepts

1. conduct disorder
2. 50 percent
3. childhood
4. normative
5. thinking
6. in the classroom
7. unintentional
8. difficult
9. false
10. underestimate
11. false
12. leaving a parent
13. rejected
14. developmental
15. aptitude; achievement
16. ADHD; oppositional defiant disorder
17. false
18. causes of
19. enuresis
20. overinclusive
21. false
22. overlapping
23. boys; women
24. internalising; externalising
25. externalising
26. suicide
27. easier
28. neglectful
29. reinforcing
30. false
31. result
32. anxiety
33. true
34. emotionally
35. false
36. self
37. true
38. depression
39. false
40. false
41. true
42. false
43. false
44. behavioural control; learning
45. true
46. false
47. true

Understanding Research

1. 4 – 16 years; hyperactivity; conduct disorder; emotional disorder (anxiety or depression); somatization disorder

2. female; teachers

3. 18 percent; less

4. boys; older; boys; somatization

5. 68 percent; within; poor; suicidal behaviour; greater

6. 50 percent; did not have a diagnosis; substance use; conduct disorder

7. convenience; children's psychological problems; A sample that is representative of the population that will be generalised to; Dewey; Truman

8. 17; 110; representative; 20; 13.4; 10; income; fewer; school

272

CHAPTER 17
ADJUSTMENT DISORDERS AND LIFE-CYCLE TRANSITIONS

Chapter Outline

I. Overview
    A. Typical Symptoms and Associated Features of Life-Cycle Transitions
    B. Classification of Life-Cycle Transitions
        1. Brief Historical Perspective
        2. Contemporary Classification of Life-Cycle Transitions

II. The Transition to Adulthood
    A. Typical Symptoms and Associated Features of the Adult Transition
        1. Identity Crisis
        2. Changes in Roles and Relationships
        3. Emotional Turmoil
    B. Classification of Identity Conflicts
    C. Epidemiology of Identity Conflicts
    D. Aetiological Considerations and Research on the Adult Transition
    E. Treatment During the Transition to Adult Life

III. Family Transitions
    A. Typical Symptoms and Associated Features of Family Transitions
        1. Family Conflict
        2. Emotional Distress
        3. Cognitive Conflicts
    B. Classification of Troubled Family Relationships
    C. Epidemiology of Family Transitions
    D. Aetiological Considerations and Research on Family Transitions
        1. Psychological Factors
            a. Communication Problems
            b. Family Roles
        2. Social Factors
        3. Biological Factors
    E. Treatment During Family Transitions
        1. Prevention Programs
        2. Couples Therapy and Family Therapy
            a. Behavioural Marital Therapy
            b. Treating Individual Problems with Couples Therapy or Family Therapy

IV. Aging and the Transition to Later Life
    A. Ageism
    B. Typical Symptoms and Associated Features of Aging
        1. Physical Functioning and Health

a. Menopause
b. Sensation and Physical Movement
2. Life Satisfaction, Work, and Relationships
a. Integrity versus Despair
b. Relationships
3. Grief and Bereavement
4. Mental Health
C. Classification of Aging
D. Epidemiology of Aging
E. Aetiological Considerations and Research on the Aging Transition
F. Treatment of Psychological Problems in Later Life

Learning Objectives

After reviewing the material presented in this chapter, you should be able to:

1. Define life-cycle transition.

2. Understand that life-cycle transitions may play a role in the development of psychopathology.

3. Describe Erikson's psychosocial moratorium and identity crisis.

4. Define Marcia's four identity statuses.

5. Describe some common gender differences that occur in the transition to adulthood.

6. Identify ways in which power struggles, intimacy struggles, affiliation, interdependence, and scapegoating impact upon the family structure.

7. Describe Gottman's four ommunication problems, giving examples for each type of problem.

8. Describe some premarital and marital therapy treatment programs.

9. Compare Bowlby's and Kubler-Ross's model of grieving in bereavement

10. Identify typical psychological and physiological processes in young-old, old-old, and oldest-old adults.

11. Describe some gender differences in adults in later life in terms of relationships.

Key Terms — Matching #1

The following terms related to adjustment disorders and difficult life events are important to know. To test your knowledge, match the following terms with their definitions. Answers are listed at the end of the chapter.

a.   Adjustment disorders
b.   Life-span development
c.   Life-cycle transitions
d.   Transition to adult life
e.   Family transitions
f.   Transition to later life
g.   Interpersonal diagnoses
h.   Crisis of the healthy personality
i.   Identity
j.   Identity versus role confusion

k.   Identity crisis
l.   Intimacy versus self-absorption
m.   Generativity versus stagnation
n.   Integrity and despair
o.   Family life cycle
p.   Early adult transition
q.   Midlife transition
r.   Late adult transition
s.   Social clocks

1.   ____   the challenge in establishing intimate relationships, balanced between closeness and independence
2.   ____   clinically significant symptoms in response to stress that are not severe enough to warrant classification as another mental disorder
3.   ____   career and family accomplishments with purpose or direction versus lacking purpose or direction
4.   ____   struggles in the process of moving from one social or psychological stage of adult development into a new one
5.   ____   a series of normal conflicts related to change as the comfortable and pre-dictable conflicts with the fearsome but exciting unknown
6.   ____   becoming less driven by internal and external demands and developing more compassion for ourselves and others
7.   ____   classification of psychological problems that reside within the context of human relationships rather than within an individual
8.   ____   age-related goals for ourselves
9.   ____   a period of basic uncertainty about self
10. ____   the challenge of adolescence and young adulthood, this stage involves integrating various role identities into a global sense of self
11. ____   fluctuations in behavior from infancy through the last years of life
12. ____   looking back on one's life with either a sense of acceptance and pride or anger and despair
13   ____   global sense of self
14. ____   the changing roles and relationships of later life
15. ____   the developmental course of family relationships throughout life
16. ____   in the middle years of life; includes birth of first child and divorce
17. ____   in the late teens and early twenties; struggling with identity, career, and relationship issues

18. _____ moving away from family and assuming adult roles
19. _____ major changes in life roles like retirement, grief over death of loved ones, and aging and facing mortality

Key Terms — Matching #2

The following terms related to adjustment disorders and difficult life events are important to know. To test your knowledge, match the following terms with their definitions. Answers are listed at the end of the chapter.

1. Moratorium
2. Identity diffusion
3. Identity foreclosure
4. Identity moratorium
5. Identity achievement
6. Alienated identity achievement
7. Empty nest
8. Power struggles
9. Intimacy struggles
10. Boundaries
11. Reciprocity
12. Demand and withdrawal pattern
13. Gene-environment correlation
14. Rational suicide
15. Scapegoat
16. Heritability
17. Heritability ratio
18. Criticism
19. Contempt
20. Defensiveness
21. Stonewalling
22. Androgynous couples
23. Behavioural marital therapy
24. Assisted suicide

a. _____ an elderly adult choosing to end their life
b. _____ couples in which both husbands and wives have high levels of masculinity and femininity
c. _____ the adjustment that occurs when adult children leave the family home
d. _____ a new identity status common in the 1960s, where one's definition of self is alienated from many values held by the larger society
e. _____ attacking someone's personality rather than his or her actions
f. _____ emphasizes the couple's moment-to-moment interaction, focusing on exchange of positive and negative behaviors, style of communication, and strategies for problem-solving
g. _____ where the wife becomes increasingly demanding and the husband withdraws further and further as time passes
h. _____ a statistic used for summarizing the genetic contributions to behavioral characteristics; equal to the variance due to genetic factors divided by the total variance in a behavioural characteristic
i. _____ the category of being in the middle of an identity crisis and actively searching for adult roles
j. _____ a form of self-justification, such as denying responsibility or blaming the other person
k. _____ social exchange of cooperation and conflict
l. _____ a pattern of isolation and withdrawal

m.	_____	attempts to change dominance relations
n.	_____	a time of uncertainty about self and goals
o.	_____	a family member who is held to blame for all of a family's troubles
p.	_____	attempts to alter the degree of closeness in a relationship
q.	_____	the category of having questioned childhood identity but not actively searching for new adult roles
r.	_____	a nonrandom association between inborn characteristics and environmental experience
s.	_____	the category of having questioned one's identity and having successfully decided on long-term goals
t.	_____	an insult motivated by anger and intended to hurt the other person
u.	_____	the rules of a relationship
v.	_____	the relative contribution of genes to behavioural characteristics
w.	_____	the category of having never questioned oneself or one's goals but instead proceeding along the predetermined course of one's childhood commitments
x.	_____	a medical professional helping a disabled person end their life

Key Terms — Matching #3

The following terms related to adjustment disorders and difficult life events are important to know. To test your knowledge, match the following terms with their definitions. Answers are listed at the end of the chapter.

a.	Ageism		j.	Obsessive reminiscence
b.	Menopause		k.	Narrative reminiscence
c.	Estrogen		l.	Grief
d.	Hormone replacement therapy		m.	Bereavement
e.	Reminiscence		n.	Gerontology
f.	Integrative reminiscence		o.	Young-old adults
g.	Instrumental reminiscence		p.	Old-old adults
h.	Transitive reminiscence		q.	Oldest-old adults
i.	Escapist reminiscence		r.	Behavioural gerontology

1.	_____	the cessation of menstruation
2.	_____	descriptive rather than interpretive
3.	_____	misconceptions and prejudices about aging
4.	_____	the recounting of personal memories of the distant past
5.	_____	the multidisciplinary study of aging
6.	_____	a female sex hormone that fluctuates during menopause
7.	_____	the emotional and social process of coping with a separation or loss
8.	_____	adults ages 85 and older
9.	_____	an attempt to achieve a sense of self-worth, coherence, and reconciliation with the past

10. ____ preoccupation with failure; full of guilt, bitterness, and despair
11. ____ adults roughly between the ages of 65 and 75; those in good health and active in their communities
12. ____ a subdiscipline of health psychology and behavioural medicine which focuses on the study and treatment of behavioural components of health and illness among older adults
13. ____ a specific form of grieving in response to the death of a loved one
14. ____ the administration of artifical estrogen
15. ____ full of glorification of the past and deprecation of the present
16. ____ includes both direct moral instruction and storytelling with clear moral implications; serves the function of passing on cultural heritage and personal legacy
17. ____ adults roughly between the ages of 75 and 85; those who suffer from major physical, psychological, or social problems and require some routine assistance in living
18. ____ the review of goal-directed activities and attainments reflecting a sense of control and success in overcoming life's obstacles

Names You Should Know — Matching

The following people have played an important role in research and theory of adjustment disorders and difficult life transitions. To test your knowledge, match the following names with the descriptions of their contributions to the study of abnormal psychology. Answers are listed at the end of the chapter.

a. Erik Erikson   c. Karen Horney   e. John Gottman
b. Daniel Levinson   d. Elisabeth Kubler-Ross

1. ____ theorized that people have competing needs to move toward, to move away from, and to move against others
2. ____ widened the emphasis of adult development to social as well as psychological tasks
3. ____ developed a stage theory of grieving in bereavement
4. ____ developed a stage theory of psychosocial development from birth to death
5. ____ focused on communication patterns in marital interaction

Review of Concepts — Fill in the Blank and True/False

This section will help focus your studying by testing whether you understand the concepts presented in the text. After you have read and reviewed the material, test your comprehension and memory by filling in the following blanks or circling the right answer. Answers are listed at the end of the chapter.

1. The DSM-IV has a comprehensive, detailed section on adjustment disorders and other conditions besides mental disorders that may be the focus of psychotherapy:

    true   false

2. Erikson focused more on the _____ side of "psychosocial" development, while Levinson focused more on the _____ aspects.

3. Research has shown that **adolescents** or **adults** experience more intense emotions.

4. The development of identity has been **focused on** or **neglected** by researchers.

5. The "forgotten half" refers to youth who do not _____.

6. Research suggests that the most successful young adults have parents who strike a balance between continuing to provide support and _____ and allowing their children increasing _____.

7. For women in traditional roles, identity often develops out of _____.

8. Marital satisfaction **increases** or **decreases** following the birth of the first child.

9. Family members with happy relationships _____ negative comments and _____ positive ones.

10. Research shows that men but not women experience high emotional arousal as _____.

11. About _____ of all existing marriages will end in divorce.

12. Divorce is likely to be followed by remarriage or a common-law relationship.

    true   false

13. Androgynous couples had marriages that were **higher** or **lower** in satisfaction than nonandrogynous couples.

14. Research indicates that the Premarital Relationship Enhancement Program **is** or **is not** effective in increasing marital satisfaction over time.

15. Behavioral marital therapy has been shown to be more effective than other therapy approaches: **true   false**

16. Couples therapy can be effective in alleviating a person's depression: **true   false**

17. **Men** or **women**   have a shorter life expectancy.

18. Older people are less satisfied with their lives: **true   false**

19. Personality has been found to be consistent from middle age to old age: **true   false**

20. Physical activity and physical health are some of the best predictors of psychological well-being among older adults: **true   falsee**

21. Hormone replacement therapy increases the risk for cancer: **true   false**

22. Visual acuity actually increases with age: **true   false**

23. Older adults report fewer positive relationships and a declined sense of mastery over their environment than young and middle age adults: **true   false**

24. Researchers have found support for the stages of bereavement proposed by Kubler-Ross: **true   false**

25. Less intense bereavement predicts better long-term adjustment: **true   false**

26. The prevalence of mental disorders increases with age: **true   false**

27. The risk of completed suicide is higher among the elderly: **true   false**

28. Men apparently benefit more from _____ while women benefit more from _____.

Multiple Choice Questions

The following multiple choice questions will test your comprehension of the material presented in the chapter. Answers are listed at the end of the chapter.

1) The divorce rates are highest in:

   a. the early years of marriage
   b. the later years of marriage
   c. between 10 and 20 years of marriage
   d. divorces rates are not related to number of years married

2) Which of the following groups has the highest suicide rate?

   a. teenagers
   b. young adults
   c. middle-aged adults
   d. adults over the age of 80

3) Which of the following includes various struggles in the process of moving from one social or psychological "stage" of adult development into a new stage?

   a. life cycle transitions
   b. transition to adult life
   c. developmental tasks of adult life
   d. family transitions

4) Approximately _____ of couples seen in behavioural marital therapy do not improve significantly.

   a. 30 percent
   b. 40 percent
   c. 50 percent
   d. 60 percent

5) According to Erikson, which of the following stages is the major challenge of adolescence and young adulthood?

   a. integrity versus despair
   b. generativity versus stagnation
   c. intimacy versus self-absorption
   d. identity versus role confusion

6) On the average, marital happiness declines following _____.

   a. the death of a family member
   b. the birth of the first child
   c. the emptying of the family nest
   d. the fifth year of marriage

7) Which of the following refers to youth who do not attend college and who often assume marginal roles in U.S. society?

   a. "Transient Youth"
   b. "Generation X"
   c. "Alienated Youth"
   d. "Forgotten Half"

8) When reviewing the various models of adult development, which of the following must be taken into consideration?

   a. that history, culture, and personal values influence views about which kinds of "tasks" are normal during adult development
   b. that transitions or "crises" may not be as predictable as the models imply
   c. some people may not pass through a particular stage of development
   d. all of the above

9) Research indicates that depression is more closely linked to _____ for women, while it is more closely liked to _____ for men.

   a. marital conflict; divorce
   b. divorce; marital conflict
   c. poor support system; financial difficulties
   d. financial difficulties; poor support system

10) The ratio of men to women _____ at older ages.

   a. increases
   b. decreases
   c. is approximately equal
   d. stays relatively the same across the age span

11) Erik Erikson highlighted _____ as a common theme that occurs throughout life cycle transitions.

   a. uncertainty   c. remorse
   b. conflict   d. acceptance

12) Estimates indicate that about _____ of all of today's marriages will end in divorce.

   a. 30 percent   c. 50 percent
   b. 40 percent   d. 60 percent

13) Epidemiological evidence indicates that the prevalence of mental disorders is _____ among adults 65 years of age and older as compared to younger adults.

   a. lower
   b. higher
   c. about the same
   d. it is unknown due to the difficulty in studying this population

14) Which of the following identifies people who are in the middle of an identity crisis and who are actively searching for adult roles?

   a. alienated identity achievement
   b. identity moratorium
   c. identify diffusion
   d. identity foreclosure

15) All of the following are emphasized by behavioral marital therapy EXCEPT:

   a. the couple's moment-to-moment interactions
   b. strategies for solving problems

c. extensive clinical interview of relationship patterns in the couple's families

d. the couple's style of communication

16) Family life cycle theorists classify adult development according to which of the following?

 a. the tasks and transitions of family life
 b. the adult's memories of their childhood and adolescence
 c. the tasks and transitions of psychological challenges of adulthood
 d. all of the above

17) Psychological research suggests that the most successful young adults have which kind of parents?

 a. parents who are strict and authoritarian
 b. parents who are supportive and could be characterized as their children's "best friend"
 c. parents who strongly encourage individuation and provide opportunities for their children to take on numerous responsibilities at an early age
 d. parents who strike a balance between continuing to provide support and supervision of their children while allowing them increasing independence

18) Which of the following individuals theorized that people have competing needs to move toward, to move away from, and to move against others?

 a. Erik Erikson   c. Karen Horney
 b. Daniel Levinson   d. Elisabeth Kubler-Ross

19) _____ struggles are attempts to change dominance relations, whereas _____ struggles are attempts to alter the degree of closeness in a relationship.

 a. Intimacy; power   c. Conflict; relational
 b. Power; intimacy   d. Relational; conflict

20) A study of adults over the age of 70 found that both men and women listed which of the following as the most common contribution to a negative quality of life in their later years?

 a. poor health   c. financial difficulties
 b. death of a spouse   d. interpersonal problems

21) All of the following are true of the "V codes" in the DSM-IV EXCEPT:

 a. they do not include an extensive summary of life difficulties
 b. they are similar to other diagnoses in the DSM in that they are diagnosed as mental disorders
 c. they include issues such as bereavement, identity problems, and phase of life problems.
 d. all of the above are true of "V codes"

22) Lisa and Mike have been married for four years. Recently, they have been arguing more than usual. Whenever they get into an argument, Lisa engages in a pattern of isolation and withdrawal, ignoring Mike's complaints and virtually ceasing all communication with him. According to the four basic communication problems identified by John Gottman, Lisa is engaged in which of the following?:

a. stonewalling
b. contempt

c. defensiveness
d. criticism

23) According to your text, all of the following are true of hormone replacement therapy EXCEPT:

a. it alleviates some of the psychological strains associated with adverse physical symptoms of menopause
b. reduces the subsequent risk for heart and bone disease
c. increases the risk for cancer
d. decreases symptoms of depression, which are often associated with menopause

24) One criticism of Erikson's theories is:

a. the stages are inappropriate for certain developmental levels
b. the theories are too broad and general and are not applicable to a large proportion of the population
c. they are not very accurate in outlining developmental stages
d. the theories focus on men to the exclusion of women

25) According to Canadian psychologists Paul Wong and Lisa Watt, which of the following is associated with less successful adjustment in later life?

a. obsessive reminiscence
b. transitive reminiscence

c. instrumental reminiscence
d. integrative reminiscence

26) Family therapists and family researchers often blame difficulties in negotiating family transitions on which of the following?

a. low motivation
b. problems with communication

c. difficulty identifying problem areas
d. all of the above

27) Which of the following is NOT a stage of adult development in Erikson's model?

a. intimacy versus self-absorption
b. integrity versus despair

c. assurance versus apprehension
d. generativity versus stagnation

28) Research on identity achievement indicates that _____ may have rejecting and distant families, while _____ may have overprotective families.

a. identity diffusers; identity foreclosers
b. identity foreclosers; identity diffusers

c. identity achievers; alienated identity achievers

d. alienated identity achievers; identity achievers

29) All of the following are stages included in the Family Developmental Tasks through the Family Life Cycle EXCEPT:

a. childbearing

b. launching center

c. aging family members

d. death and dying

Understanding Research — Fill in the Blank

The Heritability of Divorce: The text presents a detailed description of a study by McGue and Lykken in the Research Close-Up. Finding the answers to these questions will help you get a good understanding of this study and why it is important. It is not necessary to memorize the answers; the process of finding them in the textbook will help you learn the material you need to know.

1. Behavior geneticists have increasingly emphasized that people make their own

_____. Some people are risk _____ who con-

stantly seek thrills, while others are risk-_____ who seek stable, pre-

dictable environments. Family transitions may be partially determined by a person's

_____, which may be influenced by _____ factors. In

this sense, _____ may be genetic. The sample in this study includ-

ed more than _____ MZ and DZ twin pairs. MZ twins with divorced co-twins

were more than _____ times as likely to be divorced as MZ twins with

never-divorced _____. For DZ twins, the risk was less than _____

times higher if the co-twin was divorced than if the co-twin was never divorced.

The heritability of divorce was calculated at _____.

2. Clearly, there is no divorce _____. Since divorce does not occur at random,

children from divorced and married families differ in more ways than

_____. Over the past hundred years, divorce

rates have gone from _____ to _____. Environmental _____ can

eliminate or increase divorce. Therefore, the issue is genes _____ environment.

As well as personality traits, physical _____ or age at

_____ may be factors. People may find divorce more

_____ if their identical versus fraternal twin has

been divorced.

285

The Concept of Heritability: The text discusses this type of research in the Research Methods section. Finding the answers to these questions will help you get a good understanding of these issues.

3.   The _____ is the most common method used in behaviour genetics. Environmental factors are implicated in the aetiology of a disorder when the concordance rate for MZ twins is _____. Why do some experts view the heritability ratio as representing a false dichotomy?

_____

4.   Heritability estimates do not reflect the range of environments that are theoretically _____. If everyone had an identical environment, then all differences between people would be caused by _____. _____ may matter more than we are able to detect in contemporary research.

Brief Essay

As a final exercise, write out answers to the following brief essay questions. Then compare your answers with the material presented in the text.

After you have answered these questions, review the "critical thinking" questions that are presented at the end of the text chapter. Answering these questions will help you integrate important issues and themes that have been featured throughout the chapter.

1.   Discuss the stages of Erik Erikson's model of adult development. What do you consider to be the strengths of this model? What are some of its weaknesses?

2.   Outline the psychological, social, and biological factors that may contribute to difficulties in family transitions. Which factors do you think are most important when identifying the aetiology of family transition difficulties?

3.   Review the six categories of reminiscence identified by Paul Wong and Lisa Watt. Which categories appear to be related to successful aging? Which appear to be associated with less successful adjustment in later life? Which category do you think will best describe your reminiscence later in life? Why?

4.   Discuss the various categories of identity conflicts as presented in your text. Presently, which category do you fit best in? Why?

ANSWER KEY

Key Terms — Matching #1

1. l	11. b
2. a	12. n
3. m	13. i
4. c	14. r
5. h	15. o
6. q	16. e
7. g	17. d
8. s	18. p
9. k	19. f
10. j	

Names You Should Know

1. c
2. b
3. d
4. a
5. e

Key Terms — Matching #2

a. 14	m. 8
b. 22	n. 1
c. 7	o. 15
d. 6	p. 9
e. 18	q. 2
f. 23	r. 13
g. 12	s. 5
h. 17	t. 19
i. 4	u. 10
j. 20	v. 16
k. 11	w. 3
l. 21	x. 24

Key Terms - Matching #3

1. b	10. j
2. k	11. o
3. a	12. r
4. e	13. m
5. n	14. d
6. c	15. i
7. l	16. h
8. q	17. p
9. f	18. g

Multiple Choice

1. a	6. b	11. b	16. a	21. b	27. b
2. d	7. d	12. b	17. d	22. a	28. c
3. a	8. d	13. a	18. c	23. d	29. a
4. c	9. a	14. b	19. b	25. d	30. d
5. d	10. b	15. c	20. a	26. a	

Review of Concepts

1. false
2. psychological; social
3. adolescents
4. neglected
5. attend college
6. supervision; independence
7. relationships
8. decreases
9. ignore; reciprocate
10. negative

11. 40%	20. true
12. true	21. true
13. higher	22. false
14. is	23. false
15. false	24. false
16. true	25. true
17. men	26. false
18. false	27. true
19. true	28. marriage; happy relationships

Understanding Research

1. environments; takers; adverse; personality; genetic; divorce; 1,500; six; probands; two; .525

2. gene; their parents' marital status; zero; 50 percent; thresholds; and; attractiveness; marriage; socially acceptable

3. twin study; less than 100 percent; because all behaviour is the product of genes *and* environment

4. possible; genetics; Environments

CHAPTER 18
MENTAL HEALTH AND THE LAW

Chapter Outline

I. Overview

II. Mental Health, Criminal Responsibility, and Procedural Rights
  A. Mental Disorder and Criminal Responsibility
    1. M'Naghten Test
    2. Irresistible Impulse Test
    3. Not Criminally Responsible on Account of a Mental Disorder (NCRAMD)
    4. Burden of Proof
    5. Legal Definitions of Mental Disorder: Broad vs. Narrow
    6. Mental Health Professionals as Expert Witnesses
    7. Use and Consequences of Mental Disorder Defence
  B. Criminal Proceedings and Fitness to Stand Trial

III. Mental Health and Civil Law
  A. Libertarianism versus Paternalism in Treating Patients Who Have Mental Disorders
  C. Civil Commitment
    1. Grounds and Procedures
    2. Assessing Dangerousness to Self and Others
      a. Clinical Assessment and the prediction of Dangerous behaviour
      b. Assessing Suicide Risk
  D. The Rights of Patients with Mental Disorders
  E. Deinstitutionalisation
    1. The Case for Paternalism

IV. Mental Health and Family Law
  A. Children, Parents, and the State
  B. Child Custody Disputes
    1. Expert Witnesses in Custody Determinations
    2. Divorce Mediation
  C. Child Abuse

V. Professional Responsibilities and the Law
  A. Professional Negligence and Malpractice
    1. Informed Consent on the Efficacy of Alternative Treatments
    2. Who is the Client?
  B. Confidentiality
    1. Tarasoff and the Duty to Protect Potential Victims

Learning Objectives

After reviewing the material presented in this chapter, you should be able to:

1. Understand the legal and psychological definitions of mental disorder and the difference between them.

2. Describe the conditions under which mental disability limits criminal responsibility.

3. Distinguish the M'Naghten test, the irresistible impulse test, the product test, for determining insanity.

4. Know the basic statistics surrounding the use of the NCRMD plea and compare the consequences given the verdict of NCRMD with that of a "guilty" verdict

5. Understand the difference between the NGRI and NCRMD pleas and the reasons for the changes made to the Criminal Code of Canadian regarding these two sentences.

6. Understand the role of psychologists as expert witnesses in the legal system.

7. Understand the issue of "fitness to stand trial" and the role it plays in the legal system.

8. Contrast the libertarian position with that of the paternalist position regarding involuntary psychiatric commitment to an inpatient hospital.

9. Understand the reasons for the unreliaility of dangerousness predictions and suicide risk predictions.

10. Describe the basic issues involved in the psychiatric patient's right to treatment, the right to the least restrictive alternative environment, and the right to refuse treatment.

11. Know some of the problems associated with the deinstitutionalisation movement in psychiatry.

12. Describe the role of mental health practitioners in child custody disputes.

13. Delineate some of the most common types of malpractice cases that are filed against mental health practitioners.

14. List some situations in which psychologists are legally bound to break confidentiality.

Key Terms — Matching #1

The following terms related to mental health and the law are important to know. To test your knowledge, match the following terms with their definitions. Answers are listed at the end of the chapter.

a. Battle of the experts
b. Criminal responsibility
c. Civil Commitment
d. Insanity
e. Mental disorder defence
f. M'Naghten test
g. Not guilty by reason of insanity
h. Irresistible impulse test
i. Deterrence
j. Product test
k. Not Criminally responsible on account of mental disorder (NCRMD)
l. Burden of proof
m. Standard of proof
n. Expert witnesses

o. Battered woman syndrome
p. Temporary insanity
q. Fitness to Stand Trial
r. The "right from wrong" principle
s. Emergency procedures
t. Deinstitutionalisation movement
u. Libertarian
v. Paternalist
w. Preventive detention
x. Formal procedures
y. Parens patriae
z. Police power
aa. Outpatient commitment
bb. Munchausen-by-Proxy syndrome

1. ____ the inability by a defendant, on account of mental disorder, to conduct a defence at any stage of the proceedings or to instruct counsel to do so
2. ____ a legal term referring to a defendent's state of mind while committing a crime
3. ____ the state as parent
4. ____ specialists who are allowed to testify about specific matters of opinion that lie within their area of expertise
5. ____ a person being held accountable when he or she breaks the law
6. ____ the attempt to care for the mentally ill in their communities
7. ____ when different mental health experts disagree about whether a given defendant has a mental disorder
8. ____ the view that emphasises the state's duty to protect its citizens
9. ____ confinement before a crime is committed
10. ____ the psychological effects of being chronically abused by a husband or lover
11. ____ the temporary confinement of an acutely disturbed individual into a psychiatric hospital, typically for no more than a few days
12. ____ the principle for determining insanity of whether the person is prevented from knowing the wrongfulness of his or her actions by a mental disease or defect
13. ____ the stress of an event temporarily causes a person to be legally insane
14. ____ the idea that an accused person is not criminally responsible if his or her unlawful act was the product of a mental disease or defect
15. ____ involuntary hospitalisation for longer periods of time and ordered by a court
16. ____ a rule for determining insanity for a "not guilty by reason of insanity" plea
17. ____ the legal process of sending someone to a psychiatric hospital against his or her will
18. ____ the idea that people will avoid committing crimes because they fear being punished for them
19. ____ the degree of certainty required

20. ____ the principle that people could be found insane if they were unable to control their actions because of a mental disease
21. ____ the view that emphasises protecting the rights of the individual
22. ____ whether the prosecution or the defence has the obligation to prove guilt
23. ____ an attempt to prove that a person with a mental illness did not meet the legal criteria for sanity at the time of committing a crime
24. ____ the finding by a court that a person is not criminally responsible for his or her actions because of a mental disease or defect
25. ____ the state's duty to protect the public safety, health, and welfare
26. ____ a defence that entails the recognition that the person is guilty of committing the crime, but also acknowledges that the offence occurred under circumstances of a mental disorder
27. ____ a form of child abuse in which a parent feigns or induces illness in a child
28. ____ the patient is court-ordered to attend treatment

Key Terms — Matching #2

The following terms related to mental health and the law are important to know. To test your knowledge, match the following terms with their definitions. Answers are listed at the end of the chapter.

1. Base rates
2. Sensitivity
3. Specificity
4. Informed consent
5. Substituted judgement
6. Revolving door phenomenon
7. Child custody
8. Physical custody
9. Legal custody
10. Sole custody
11. Joint custody
12. Mediator
13. Child's best interests standard
14. Divorce mediation
15. Child abuse
16. Physical child abuse
17. Child sexual abuse
18. Child neglect
19. Psychological abuse
20. Foster care
21. Professional responsibilities
22. Negligence
23. Malpractice
24. Confidentiality

a. ____ where the children will live at what times
b. ____ population frequencies
c. ____ repeated denigration in the absence of physical harm
d. ____ a legal decision that involves determining where children will reside and how parents will share legal rights and responsibilities for child rearing
e. ____ the ethical obligation not to reveal private communications
f. ____ a neutral third party who facilitates the parents' discussions
g. ____ more patients are admitted to psychiatric hospitals more frequently but for shorter periods of time

h. _____ parents meet with a neutral third party who helps them to identify, negotiate, and resolve their disputes during a divorce

i. _____ a temporary placement of the child outside of his or her home

j. _____ appointing an independent guardian to provide informed consent when a person is not competent to provide it for himself or herself

k. _____ when professional negligence results in harm to patients

l. _____ the standard that governs custody disputes

m. _____ how the parents will make separate or joint decisions about their children's lives

n. _____ true positives over the sum of true positives and false negatives

o. _____ involves placing children at risk for serious physical or psychological harm by failing to provide basic and expected care

p. _____ a situation in which only one parent retains custody of the children

q. _____ involves sexual contact between an adult and child

r. _____ a situation in which both parents retain custody

s. _____ a legal decision that a parent or other responsible adult has inflicted damage or offered inadequate care to a child

t. _____ when a professional fails to perform in a manner that is consistent with the level of skill exercised by other professionals in the field

u. _____ true negatives divided by the sum of the true negatives and false positives

v. _____ involves the intentional use of physically painful and harmful actions

w. _____ a professional's obligations to meet the ethical standards of the profession and to uphold the laws of the states in which he or she practices

x. _____ the requirement that a clinician tell a patient about a procedure and its risks, the patient understands the information and freely consents to the treatment, and the patient is competent to give consent

Names You Should Know — Matching

The following people have played an important role in research and theory of mental health and the law. To test your knowledge, match the following names with the descriptions of their contributions to the study of abnormal psychology. Answers are listed at the end of the chapter.

a. Christopher Webster c. Lenore Walker
b. John Monahan d. Henry Kempe

1. _____ researched the relation between violence and mental illness, and predicting dangerousness

2. _____ wrote about the "battered child syndrome"

3. _____ A leading expert in the development of methods of risk assessment

4. _____ coined the term "the battered woman syndrome"

Review of Concepts — Fill in the Blank and True/False

This section will help focus your studying by testing whether you understand the concepts presented in the text. After you have read and reviewed the material, test your comprehension and memory by filling in the following blanks or circling the right answer. Answers are listed at the end of the chapter.

1. The legal system views abnormal behaviour very differently from the way it is understood by mental health professionals   **true**   **false**

2. Defendants are _____ if they are judged to be unable to responsibly exercise their right to participate in their own trial defence.

3. _____ is intended to protect the public and to enable the person to recover from his or her mental disorder in a safe environment.

4. The irresistible impulse test and the product test   **narrowed**   or   **broadened** the grounds for determining insanity.

5. In 1991, the Supreme Court of Canada amended the Criminal Code to give the accused persons with mental illness greater _____.

6. Some of the major changes included reductions in how long an accused person could be detained in a psychiatric facility, changes in the procedures for making appeals, and most importantly, there were changes in the mental disorder defence. The NGRI defence was changed to the _____.

7. In federal courts today, the burden of proof of a defendant's insanity lies with the **prosecution**   **defence**

8. Substance abuse lowers a psychiatric inpatient's risk of committing violence: **true**   **false**

9. The NCRMD, like the NGRI, entails automatic detention in a psychiatric hospital **true**   **false**

10. Most defendants who are found Not Guilty by Reason of Insanity spend substantially less time in a mental hospital than they would have spent in prison: **true**   **false**

11. The goal of commitment following an NGRI verdict is _____.

12. Fitness to stand trial refers to the defendant's _____ mental state and insanity refers to the defendant's state of mind at the time of _____.

13. Deinstitutionalisation refers to the movement to treat patients in _____ instead of in _____.

14. Canadian law provides for the confinement of someone who is about to commit a crime: **true**   **false**

15. What percent of the mentally disturbed have no history of violence?   _____

16. Clinicians can usually predict violence quite accurately: **true**   **false**

17. The development of resources to treat people in their communities grew rapidly with the deinstitutionalisation movement: **true**   **false**

18. Many community mental health centres do not offer services to the seriously mentally ill: **true**   **false**

19. Many patients that would have been institutionalised before are now in jail or are homeless: **true**   **false**

20. Mental health law is mostly based on the state's _____ and family law is mostly based on the state's _____.

21. Several large-scale studies have shown that divorce itself has little negative effect on children's mental health: **true**   **false**

22. Research evidence suggest that conflict between parents is strongly related to maladjustment among children following divorce: **true**   **false**

23. Mental health professionals are not permitted to break confidentiality, even to report child abuse: **true**   **false**

24. One common ground for successful malpractice suits against mental health professionals is the existence of a _____ relationship.

25. The Tarasoff case established a mental health professional's duty to _____ a potential victim of their client.

Multiple Choice Questions

The following multiple choice questions will test your comprehension of the material presented in the chapter. Answers are listed at the end of the chapter.

1) _____ commitment procedures allow an acutely disturbed individual to be temporarily confined in a mental hospital, typically for no more than a few days, while _____ commitment procedures can lead to involuntary hospitalisation that is ordered by the court and typically lasts for much longer.

    a. Formal; emergency   c. Medical; crisis
    b. Emergency; formal   d. Crisis; medical

2) All of the following have been goals of deinstitutionalisation EXCEPT:

    a. to prevent inappropriate mental hospital admissions through arranging community alternatives to treatment
    b. to release to the community all institutionalised patients who have been given adequate preparation for such a change
    c. to decrease the influx of patients by not allowing them continued access to mental hospitals and thus encouraging independence
    d. to establish and maintain community support systems for non-institutionalised people receiving mental health services in the community

3) The majority of custody decisions are made by:

    a. parents themselves
    b. attorneys who negotiate for the parents outside of court
    c. a judge and decided in court
    d. mental health professionals who evaluate the case

4) All of the following are true of the parens patriae EXCEPT:

    a. it is used to justify the state's supervision of minors and incapacitated adults
    b. it is based on the state's duty to protect the public safety, health, and welfare
    c. commitment under these rationales was virtually unknown to the United States until the early 1950s
    d. it refers to the concept of the "state as parent"

5) Following a civil commitment to a mental hospital, mental patients' rights include all of the following EXCEPT:

    a. right to treatment
    b. right to design their own treatment plan
    c. right to refuse treatment
    d. right to treatment in the least restrictive alternative environment

6) The old (NGRI) mental disorder defence was used very rarely in Canadian courts, whereas it appears that the NCRMD defence is being used somewhat more frequently. This is because:

    a. NCRMD, unlike NGRI, does not entail automatic detention in psychiatric hospital
    b. NGRI, unlike NCRMD, does not entail automatic detention in psychiatric hospital
    c. NCRMD usually results in acquital
    d. None of the above

7) All of the following stages are part of Lenore Walker's stages of the "cycle of violence" EXCEPT:

    a. battering incident   c. loving contrition
    b. tension-building phase   d. verbal reprimands

8) On the average, defendants who are found "not criminally responsible on account of mental disorder" (NCRMD) spend _____ time confined in an institution as they would have if they had been given a prison sentence instead.

    a. significantly less   c. approximately the same
    b. twice as much   d. roughly three times as much

9) Which of the following terms is defined as the ethical obligation not to reveal private communication and is basic to psychotherapy?

    a. confidentiality   c. classified information
    b. private communications   d. privileged communications

10) Mental disorders and the actions that result from them are typically viewed as:

    a. choices
    b. conditions that are outside of voluntary control
    c. responsibilities that the mentally disordered individual must assume
    d. a and c

11) All of the following are issues of special relevance regarding involuntary hospitalisation of the severely mentally impaired EXCEPT:

    a. criminal record   c. patients' rights
    b. civil commitment   d. deinstitutionalisation

12) Research indicates that approximately _____ of the mentally disturbed are not violent.

    a. 30 percent   c. 70 percent
    b. 50 percent   d. 90 percent

13) All of the following are grounds that tend to dominate commitment laws EXCEPT:

    a. being dangerous to others   c. being dangerous to self
    b. inability to care for self   d. inability to care for others

14) Over _____ of all reports of child abuse are found to be unsubstantiated after an investigation.

    a. one-eighth   c. one-half
    b. one-quarter   d. two-thirds

15) Empirical research on children's adjustment after divorce indicates that:

    a. a substantial portion of the difficulties found among children after divorce actually begins long before the marital separation occurs
    b. the psychological functioning of children from divorced families does not differ from that of children from non-divorced families
    c. the difficulties children experience are directly related to marital conflict and divorce
    d. children from divorced families tend to have more internalising problems than children from non-divorced families

16) One more common malpractice claim against mental health professionals is:

    a. the misuse of psychotherapeutic techniques
    b. the inappropriate use of electroconvulsive therapy (ECT)
    c. the failure to disclose therapeutic interpretations to clients
    d. inappropriate hospitalisation

17) Confidentiality between a therapist and a client can be broken under which of the following circumstances?

    a. the client is threatening to harm another person
    b. the client has disclosed sexual or physical abuse of a child
    c. the client is threatening to harm himself or herself
    d. all of the above

18) Which of the following is NOT TRUE of the legal definition of "fitness to stand trial competence"?

    a. it refers to the defendant's ability to understand criminal proceedings
    b. it refers to the defendant's current mental status
    c. it refers to the defendants willingness to participate in criminal proceedings
    d. the "reasonable degree" of understanding needed to establish competence is generally acknowledged to be fairly low

19) Evidence suggests that in child custody cases, mediation:

    a. does not necessarily reduce the number of custody hearings in court
    b. is more effective than the role that mental health professionals play in custody cases, and thus mental health professionals should limit their involvement in the legal system
    c. does not help parents reach decisions more quickly than if they were to go through custody hearings in court
    d. is viewed by parents as more favourable than litigation, especially fathers

20) Which of the following is TRUE regarding the idea that mental disability should limit criminal responsibility?

    a. it is a relatively new concept among mental health professionals
    b. it dates back to ancient Greek and Hebrew traditions and was evident in early English law
    c. it has emerged in our legal system within the past 50 years
    d. it surfaced following World War II when large numbers of veterans experienced post-traumatic stress symptoms and committed violent acts

21) In his research on the prediction of dangerousness, Monahan has found which of the following to be several times higher among prison inmates as among the general population?

    a. major depression   c. schizophrenia
    b. bipolar disorder   d. all of the above

Understanding Research — Fill in the Blank

The Accuracy of Predictions of Violence: The text presents a detailed description of a study by Lidz, Mulvey, and Gardner in the Research Close-Up. Finding the answers to these questions will help you get a good understanding of this study and why it is important. It is not necessary to memorise the answers; the process of finding them in the textbook will help you learn the material you need to know.

1.   Older studies on the prediction of violence were _____. This study

    examined _____ cases seen in a psychiatric _____ room

    in an urban area. Half the cases were predicted to have some

    _____ for violence by _____ clinicians who interviewed them;

    the other half were comparison cases who were not predicted to be violent.

    Patients were matched on age, sex, race, and hospital

    _____. The patient and someone that _____ them

    were later interviewed about subsequent _____ of

violence. Interviews were conducted _____ times in the _____ months following their contact with the emergency room.

2.   Investigators found that _____ percent of the predicted cases engaged in violence versus _____ percent of the comparison cases. Predictions of violence among _____ were less accurate, no better than chance, because of the clinician's underestimation of the _____. The critical distinction was the decision of whether the potential for violence was _____ or

     _____.

Base Rates and Predictions: The text discusses this research issue in the Research Methods section. Finding the answers to these questions will help you get a good understanding of these issues.

3.   The validity with which violence can be predicted depends on the

     _____ of the relation between the predictor and the outcome, and also by _____. Using a coin flip to predict violence results in a sensitivity of _____ percent, and a specificity of _____percent. With this method, the percentage of false positives is much _____. If the base rate is set at 50 percent, which would be better in the example given, the clinician's predictions or the coin flip? _____.

Brief Essay

As a final exercise, write out answers to the following brief essay questions. Then compare your answers with the material presented in the text.

   After you have answered these questions, review the "critical thinking" questions that are presented at the end of the text chapter. Answering these questions will help you integrate important issues and themes that have been featured throughout the chapter.

1.   Greg is a 35-year-old white male who was recently arrested for sexually abusing a seven-year-old girl. Although this is Greg's first offence, he has a history of "sexual addictions" that range from viewing pornography while masturbating to exhibitionism. Explain how you think criminal law would conceptualise Greg's behaviour and how you think a mental health professional would conceptualise Greg's behaviour. Discuss the similarities and differences of the two conceptualisations.

2. What are the basic underlying principles of libertarianism and paternalism? Which view do you most agree with? Defend your position.

3. Discuss the major differences between NGRI and NCRMD and the reasons why the Canadian Supreme Court adopted this latter sentence.

ANSWER KEY

Key Terms — Matching #1

1. q	11. x	21. u
2. d	12. f	22. l
3. y	13. p	23. e
4. n	14. j	24. g
5. b	15. s	25. z
6. t	16. r	26. k
7. a	17. c	27. bb
8. v	18. i	28. aa
9. w	19. m	
10. o	20. h	

Names You Should Know

1. b
2. d
3. a
4. c

Key Terms — Matching #2

a. 8	m. 19
b. 1	n. 2
c. 19	o. 18
d. 7	p. 10
e. 24	q. 17
f. 12	r. 11
g. 6	s. 15
h. 14	t. 22
i. 20	u. 3
j. 5	v. 16
k. 23	w. 21
l. 13	x. 4

Multiple Choice

1. b	7. d	13. d	19. d
2. c	8. c	14. c	20. b
3. b	9. a	15. a	21. d
4. c	10. b	16. b	
5. b	11. a	17. d	
6. a	12. d	18. c	

Review of Concepts

1. true
2. unfit to stand trial
3. detention
4. broadened
5. greater procedural and civil rights
6. not criminally responsible on account of mental disorder
7. defence
8. false
9. false
10. true
11. treatment
12. current; the crime
13. in their communities; psychiatric hospitals
14. false
15. 90 percent
16. false
17. false
18. true
19. true
20. police power; parens patriae
21. true
22. true
23. false
24. sexual
25. warn

Understanding Research

1. flawed; 714; emergency; potential; two; admission; knew; episodes; three; six

2. 53 percent; 36 percent; women; base rate; present; absent

3. magnitude; base rates; 50 percent; 50 percent; higher; coin flip

NOTES

NOTES

NOTES

NOTES